Reviews of The Low Back Yogi program

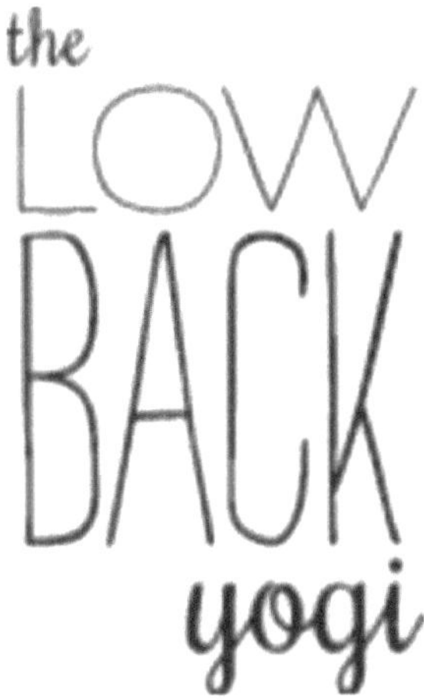

"I started going to group yoga classes a few years ago to complement my normal routine and help prevent injuries. I am quite happy to have been introduced to Justin's series, as the sequence is far more tailored to my needs. Quite usefully, Justin explains the logic behind the poses chosen, as well as the reasoning behind why you might be better off skipping some of the poses included in typical group classes. I recommend the course to anyone who has dealt with back pain in the past as well as anyone who wants to improve core strength and stability."

-Jacob Mays

"I think he did a great job of presenting the material. He focused on a specific therapy (yoga for the low back) instead of trying to teach all yoga for all body parts to everyone and that was a wonderful thing because it delivered exactly what was promised in the title of the course…He seems to CARE about the practitioners too which is nice. He gives reasons why you should do things a certain way and he gives advice as to how to approach the practice and what to do for your back pain when you're not practicing. His goal really seems to be helping people in pain. There were some non traditional moves that were new to me and that says a lot because I'm always studying exercise and constantly searching for variety. I find anyone who can inspire me with something new very refreshing!!!"

-Sky Nicholas

"This feels revolutionary. I think with continued practice this could help relieve lower back pain for many people familiar with yoga…The instructor is obviously very knowledgeable and yet also has a gentle, encouraging tone. He is a joy to watch and listen to. I don't think this course needs to be changed in any way. It does exactly what it says, and I believe it would provide great results

over time for dedicated students who proceed with the caution the instructor recommends."
-Patricia Smith

"I don't know anything about yoga but this helped me and it's one I'll watch again and again and take notes."
-Lovely L. Jones

Acknowledgments

I found the keys to solving my chronic back pain in three books written by Dr. Stu McGill: *Low Back Disorders, Ultimate Back Fitness and Performance,* and *Back Mechanic.* I would like to thank Dr. McGill for his years of dedicated research as director of the spine biomechanics lab at the University of Waterloo. I would also like to thank my many yoga students over the years who encouraged me to write this book, particularly those students who participated in the video version of this yoga course on Udemy and provided feedback. You have been instrumental to the success of the Low Back Yogi program, and I am deeply grateful for your contributions.

CHAPTER ONE

Introduction

A Yoga Teacher's Journey Out Of Yoga-Induced Back Pain

Yoga has somehow managed to get itself a great reputation for helping to improve back pain, but here's yoga's dirty little secret: most group yoga classes are absolute *murder* on the back, and can do far more harm than good in many cases.

Here's the science:

The middle of your spinal discs are made up of a liquid gel, called the nucleus, which is surrounded by rings of collagen fibers that keep the nucleus in place.

What happens when you repeatedly bend forward into spinal flexion, as you so often do in yoga poses, is that you create hydraulic pressure in the nucleus.

Every forward-bending cycle causes the collagen fibers to loosen and, over time, to slowly delaminate.

All this forward-bending produces hydraulic stress of the nucleus, posteriorly, on the fibers that are slowly delaminating.

As a result, repeated spinal flexion will slowly pump the nucleus through the delaminating collagen fibers, to create a posterior bulge in the spinal disc.

As Dr. Stu McGill has been known to say, "life isn't fair," and one's ability to withstand repeated cycles of flexion depends greatly on the discs you inherited from your parents. Some people can get away with spinal flexion for longer, and under much higher loads, than others.

As a yoga practitioner turned yoga instructor, I got away with aggressive yogic flexion exercises for about two years, feeling no ill effects. Then, when I did suddenly feel the onset of chronic back pain, it was too late. The damage had already been done.

You do not feel the delamination process happening in your spinal discs, you only feel it when it's too late, when the disc material bulges through the delaminated collagen fibers and causes nerve irritation.

If you go to a yoga class *already* experiencing low back pain, this delamination process has probably already begun — perhaps from an injury, too much sitting, aggressive exercise, etc.— and most yoga classes will only make the pain worse in the long term. If you start a yoga practice without back pain, chances are your group yoga classes will *give* you back pain if you keep at it long enough.

The confusing thing about this is that yoga stretching will *almost always* provide some short-term relief of back pain symptoms, even if the postures are exacerbating underlying structural issues. This happens because the "stretch reflex" is a neurological phenomenon that reduces pain sensitivity, but unfortunately it only lasts about 15 to 20 minutes. (See https://www.theptdc.com/2017/04/back-pain-myths/ for more from Dr. McGill on this issue.) Like most things that feel good, the pleasure we feel from stretching can make us feel like all we need is more of that feel-good-thing. But if you have back pain, the *last* thing I recommend you should do is go to a yoga class and engage in aggressive spinal-flexion and spine-twisting postures, to 'loosen up.' Chances are, you're already doing too much rounding and slouching in your day-to-day life. Going to yoga class, and rounding and twisting your spine even more, isn't going to do you any favors.

Trust me on this.

Yoga made me feel so good at first that I decided to dedicate my life to teaching it…but then, suddenly, I found that I was in so much pain that my life began to revolve around how much my back was hurting.

You'd think that suddenly having crawl to the bathroom on my hands and knees would make me re-evaluate my yoga practice, but all my teachers and gurus were telling me that yoga was 'good' for my bad back, and my whole life was tied up in yoga, so I couldn't *conceive* that it was hurting me. I just thought, "Wow, if my back is hurting this bad while I'm doing a lot of yoga, imagine how much worse it would be if I weren't doing any yoga at all!" I couldn't let in the notion that the thing I'd based my career on was actually hurting me.

Students often come to yoga thinking that if they can just 'open up,' improve their flexibility, their range of motion, they will feel relief from their 'locked-up' backs.

But what if our central nervous systems are smarter than we are? What if our back muscles are 'locking up' for a reason, to prevent us from engaging in harmful movement patterns? What if—as has been shown time and again— improved flexibility is an increased risk factor for back pain, rather than a preventative measure, as is so often assumed?

What if improved strength, stiffness and stability in our spines is what we need to lead more pain-free lives? This would fly in the face of what I like to call "Yoga Logic," which says that more flexibility is always better. But this is what the science bears out:

THE MORE 'FLEXIBLE' YOUR SPINE, THE MORE YOU ARE PUTTING YOURSELF AT RISK FOR BACK PAIN.

When it comes to most back pain, the fact is that there is **no known benefit** to greater spinal flexibility.

The research undertaken by Dr. Stu McGill's Spine Biomechanics Laboratory at the University of Waterloo has proven time and again that delaminated collagen fibers and micro-movements of the spinal joints, irritating the spinal nerves, are the prime culprits in back pain. Therefore, targeting the back muscles for yoga stretching and flexibility work *will* cause further weakness, instability, delamination and pain.

This is what happened to me.

I was able to eliminate my debilitating lower back pain, but only by quitting my group yoga practice—not to mention my yoga teaching career—and applying Dr. McGill's research and creating an individualized, home-based yoga practice for myself.

There *is* something to be said for the sense of discipline and community that one can derive from a strong group yoga experience. Unfortunately, this comes at a price: lack of personal attention, poorly-trained and/or inexperienced instructors, pre-set posture sequences that might be good for someone's bottom line but which have nothing to do with your body. The popularity and corporatization of yoga has resulted in a concomitant lack of autonomy for yoga teachers, who have been turned into trained parrots whose job it is to recite scripts, play certain music, lead people through pre-set one-size-fits-all posture sequences that have been established by a guru or a corporation. It has become a billion dollar industry built on the backs of people making poverty-level wages, resulting in high turnover. For the most part, group yoga instructors in America are under paid, under trained, and woefully ill equipped to deal with back pain patients. I have come to believe that a one-size-fits-all approach to *any* form of exercise is a recipe for disaster; for injury, re-injury, and chronic pain.

When I left my own teaching career and set my mind to creating a home yoga practice that would heal my back, I felt like I was starting from scratch. My poor yoga-abused back was hyper sensitive to forward-bending, but I also didn't do well with end-range extension (those deep, sexy back bends).
Figuring out which postures would help me rather than hurt me wasn't easy, since most yoga poses are seriously contraindicated for back pain, and I had to get past my attachment to "Yoga Logic." But, after great effort and research, I have developed a challenging yet conservative approach to yoga that eliminates most of the problematic issues that link yoga with chronic back pain.

Instead of focusing on arbitrary "flexibility," the focus of this course is on strength, endurance, stability, and *appropriate* mobility. Some areas of the body are great candidates for yoga-style mobility work—ball and socket joints like the shoulders and hips, for example— but not the spinal joints, which need to be 'locked down' in those of us with back pain.
The concepts of Beginner's Mind, forgetting everything you've been taught and think you know about yoga, and Mastery of Simplicity, which really just boils down to patience, are concepts I encourage my students to embrace.

Most rank-and-file yoga teachers mean well, but I strongly believe that for those of us with serious back problems, the only way to experience the benefits of a sensible yoga practice that will contribute to good back health, rather than wrecking it, is to establish an individualized home practice and arm ourselves with knowledge about the science of back pain.
I was afraid of my back pain for many years, because I didn't understand it. I didn't understand it because I was afraid of looking beyond the soft tissue,

afraid that if I had "disc problems" or more profound structural issues, I would wind up needing back surgery (which was not true). I also didn't understand my back pain because, for economic reasons, the science of back pain hasn't penetrated the yoga world…like, *at all*. If it ever does penetrate, yoga studios are going to have to drastically rethink their business model and teaching practices.

I'm certainly not saying that yoga is "bad!" It is simply a tool, and like any other tool it can be used well or it can be used improperly. Yoga certainly *can*, if practiced wisely, offer a path out of debilitating lower back pain. So, if you suffer from back pain and are new to the practice of yoga, I believe you've come to the right place. If you're an experienced yogi, but have been frustrated in the past with yoga's seeming inability to help you with your chronic pain, you've also come to the right place.

Together we will construct your individualized science-based yoga practice, free from the corrupting influences of dogma, ego, and a hyper-competitive fitness industrial complex; a practice rooted, fundamentally, in your body's innate wisdom.

CHAPTER TWO

How to Use This Course

Every practitioner is different, every body has different needs, and one size *never* fits all.

With that in mind, I have endeavored to provide back pain sufferers with a small handful of conservative yoga postures that can form the basis of a sensible home practice. Not all of these exercises are going to be helpful to you, and I would like you to pay close attention to your body and cherry pick only those poses that resonate with your body and leave you feeling better. Discard whatever doesn't work for you.

If you are currently in acute pain, I would encourage you to discontinue any current exercise or yoga practice, which clearly hasn't been doing you any favors.

Practice these postures at least a few times per week. I particularly recommend Dr. Stu McGill's "Big 3" Exercises—the Bird Dog, Planks, and Curl-Ups—all of which you will find in these pages.

It is only once your pain level has been significantly reduced that you'll be in a position to resume other activities and figure out which ones are pain triggers.

NOTE TO EXPERIENCED YOGIS:
If you are a regular yoga practitioner and find yourself missing the 'stretching' feeling provided by lots of bending and twisting of the spine, I recommend finding a good massage therapist who can help relieve some of that 'tightness' in your tissues *without* you having to concertina your spine into unstable, irritative positions. **Thai massage or any other modality that incorporates yoga-like back stretching should be avoided.** Acupuncture can also be helpful, as can diligent self-care with foam rollers and massage balls.

For those times when you *really* crave some yoga spinal-flexion stretching, the only pose I can wholeheartedly recommend is Cat-Camel Pose, which you will find later in this book.

The strength and stability work you'll learn in this course can certainly help with muscle pain even without aggressive stretching, because the contraction-relaxation cycles your muscles engage in when performing strength and stability work can act as a mechanism for flushing the involved muscles of metabolites (metabolic byproducts like amino acids, nucleotides and organic acids that can accumulate in the muscles due to dysfunction, robbing them of power and strength). Strength and stability work, along with occasional massage or acupuncture, are in my opinion the best methodologies for restoring proper function to muscular 'trigger points' by increasing blood flow and clearing metabolites, resulting in reduced discomfort and improved performance. However, massage and acupuncture alone—or used as 'damage control' to support a poorly-designed yoga or exercise regimen—can only provide short-term relief and will fail to address underlying weakness and the poor postural and motor control patterns that perpetuate deeper structural issues. You're just treating a symptom, not a cause. Massage and/or acupuncture combined with *appropriate* strength and mobility work is the best way to go.

Another thing you can do to support your practice and help reduce your pain level is to make certain that you're properly supporting your lumbar spine when sitting and sleeping. It's worth looking into the back supports offered on Dr. Stu McGill's website, backfitpro.com. I'm not affiliated with Dr. McGill in any way, but I've had great success with his products.

For your home practice, all you need is a yoga mat and one kettlebell.

One final thing to keep in mind is that, when incorporating kettlebells into your practice, it's vitally important that you use a *moderate* weight. The goal here is never going to be the creation of strength alone. Having a lot of strength, but very little endurance, is almost as much a risk factor for pain and injury as having a lot of 'flexibility.' Using really heavy weights robs you of the opportunity to concomitantly create *endurance* during the rehabilitation process. So for those of you who tend to want to do too much, too fast, you're going to have to rein in that ego and do less, more slowly!

The *Low Back Yogi* book and video series are designed to be used independently of one another, but if you would like to follow along with the video version of the course, you can find it at: **www.udemy.com/yoga-for-low-back-pain.**

Let's get started!

CHAPTER THREE

Braced Neutral

To begin your practice, I'd like you to start by getting a feel for the Braced Neutral Spine Position.

1. Stand with your feet shoulder width apart, toes pointing straight ahead. Now think about spreading the floor apart with your feet. Your toes aren't *actually* going to move—you're just going for the sensation of gently spreading your left foot counter-clockwise while spreading your right foot clockwise—and this sensation of 'screwing your feet into the floor' will help you activate your gluteal muscles.

2. Now I want you to poke yourself in the obliques with your fingertips.

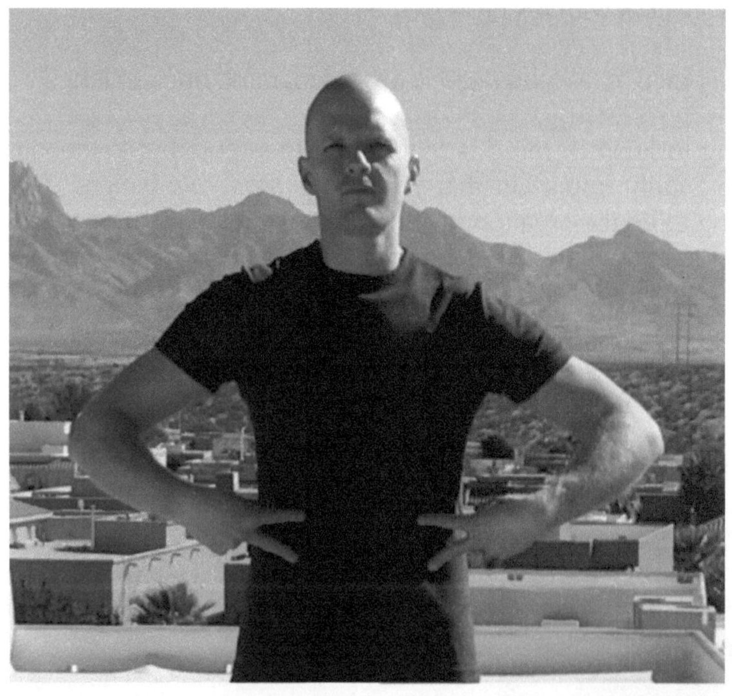

To activate your oblique muscles, all you have to do is push out against the pressure of your fingertips. Oblique activation is important in helping your body access its natural 'back brace. 'To complete the brace, tighten your abs, like someone is about to punch you in the belly. You don't need to squeeze your obliques and your abdominals as hard as you possibly can, I just want you to maintain about a 30% contraction effort. This muscular bracing is an *extremely* important component in preventing back pain.

3. Now draw your shoulder blades gently down and back, open up your chest even more.

Remember: micro-movements of the spinal joints, which irritate the spinal nerves, are a root cause of most back pain. By bracing and 'locking down' the spine we help prevent those micro-movements and reduce your pain. Mastering Braced Neutral is key to this process.

I *always* start my practice with just a few deep breaths in Braced Neutral position. It's a great way to bring mindfulness to one's overall posture, and it can translate to better postural habits in day-to-day life.

I've noticed that a lot of my back pained students have the tendency to hold their arms in front, and slouch about the head and shoulders.

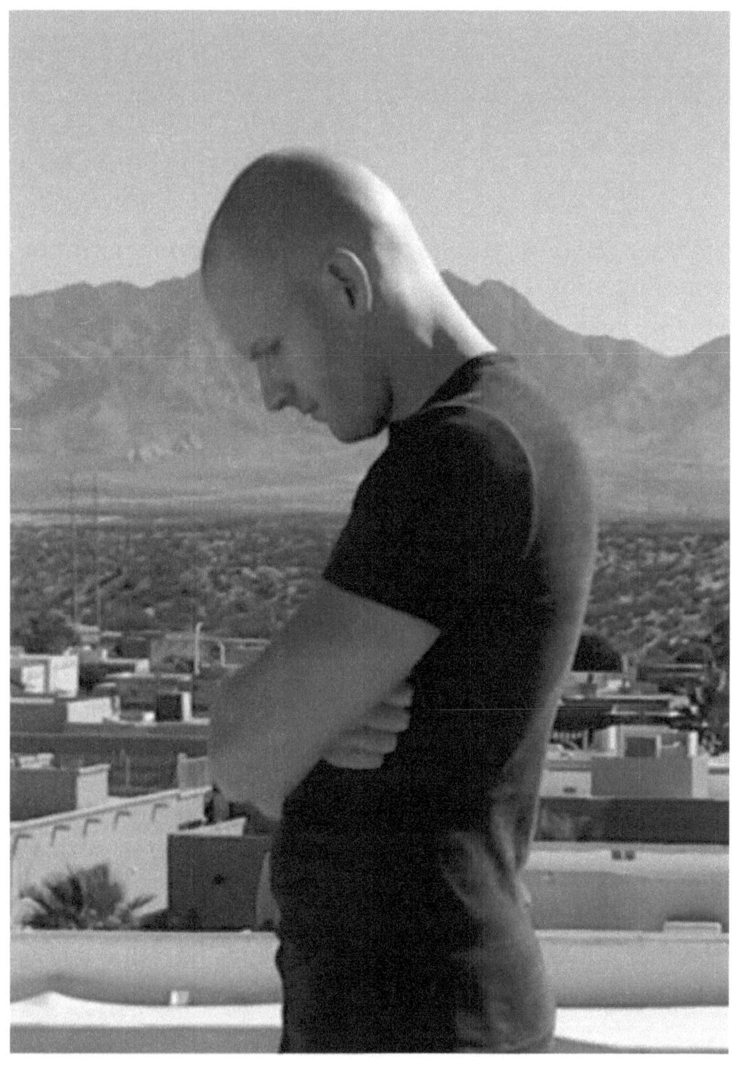

This is incredibly taxing to the spinal musculature and can contribute to your pain. Next time you catch yourself standing around and slouching like a depressed monkey, I would encourage you to stand with your head neutral, your chest open and your shoulders back.

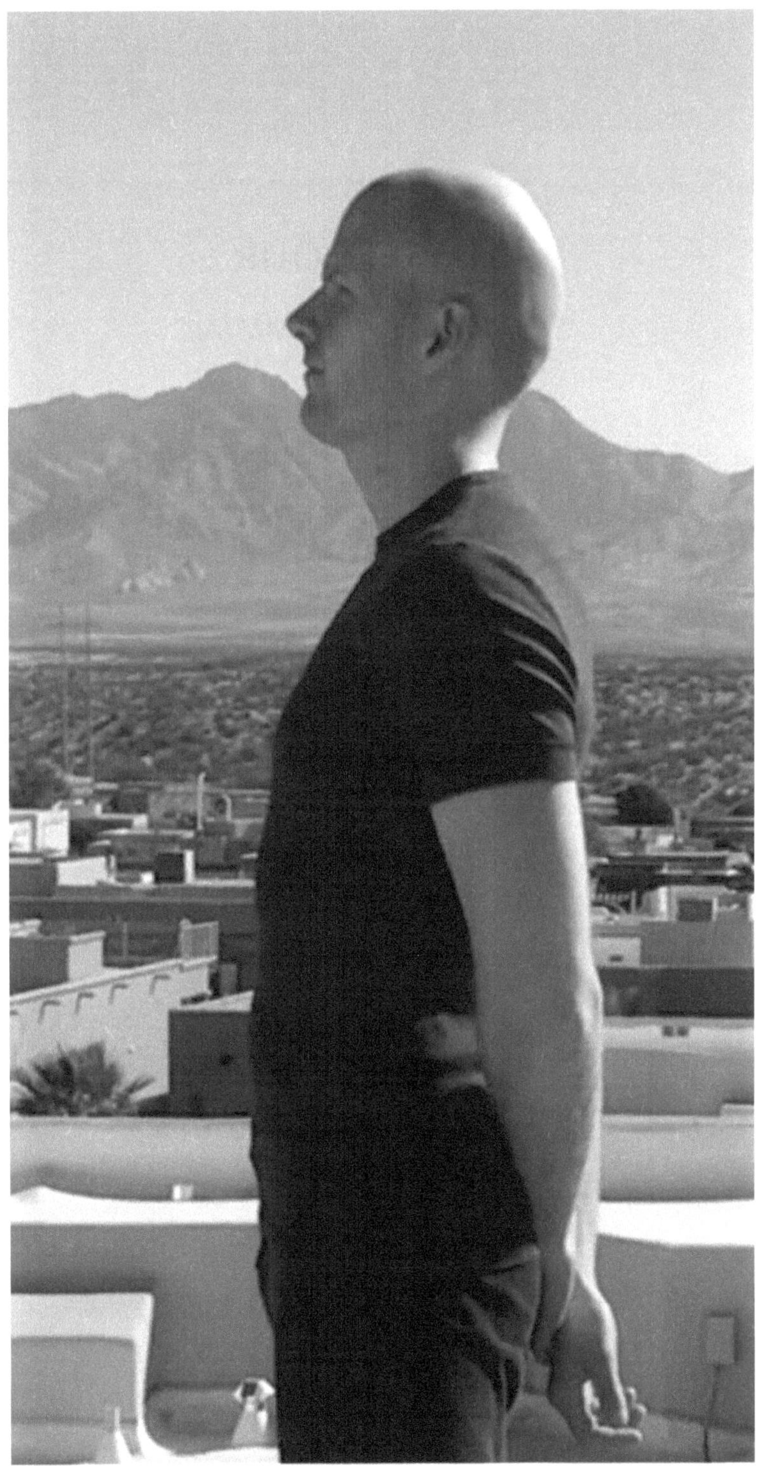

These little tweaks you make off the yoga mat can have a substantive impact on your day-to-day pain levels!

CHAPTER FOUR

Standing Deep Breathing

1. Stand in Braced Neutral Pose, then interlace your fingers just below your chin.

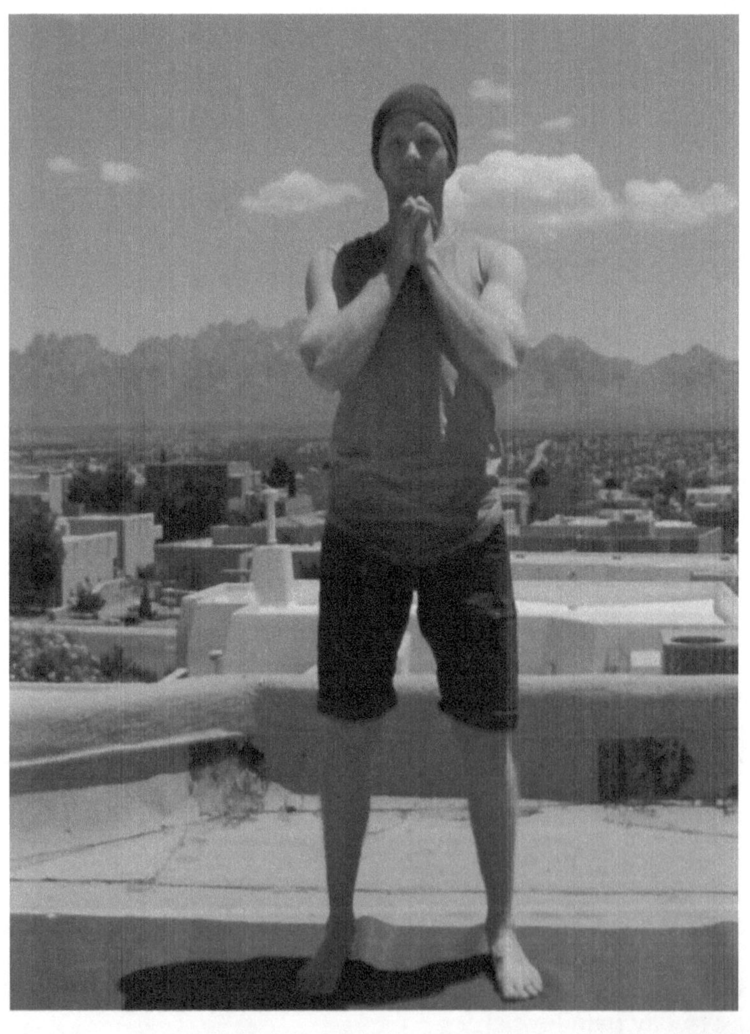

2. Inhale deeply through your nose, taking 5 or 6 seconds to fill your lungs completely, and as you inhale raise your elbows to the sky, almost like you're trying to crack your knuckles underneath your chin. It's not a contest to see how high you can get your elbows, just find a nice, natural stretch that doesn't provoke any pain.

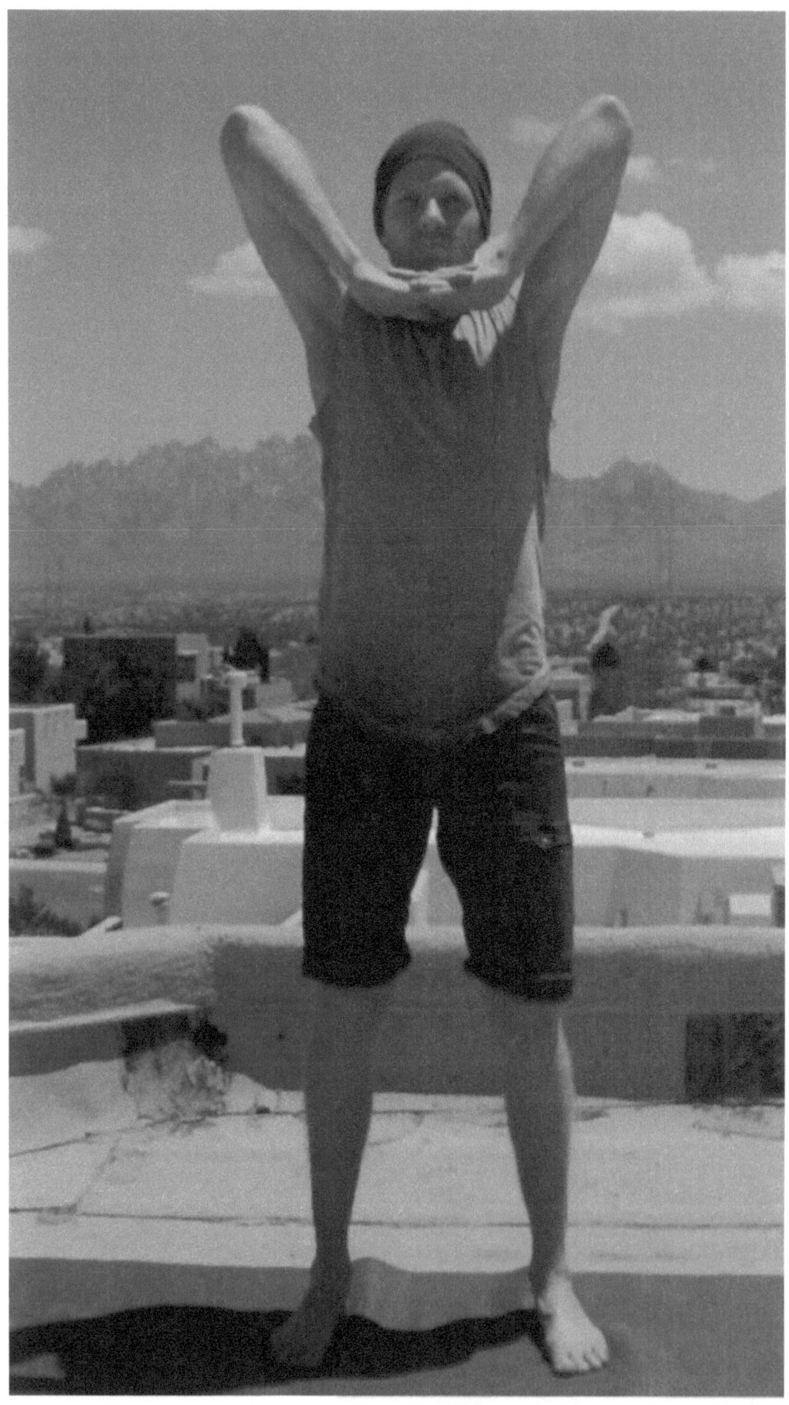

3. Take 5 or 6 seconds to fully exhale, and as you do so, tilt your head back and slowly bring your elbows together, maintaining light contact against the chin with the knuckles. If you can't tilt your head very far back or get your

elbows very close together, that's fine; just find your natural pain-free range of motion. As you keep practicing, your mobility will improve.

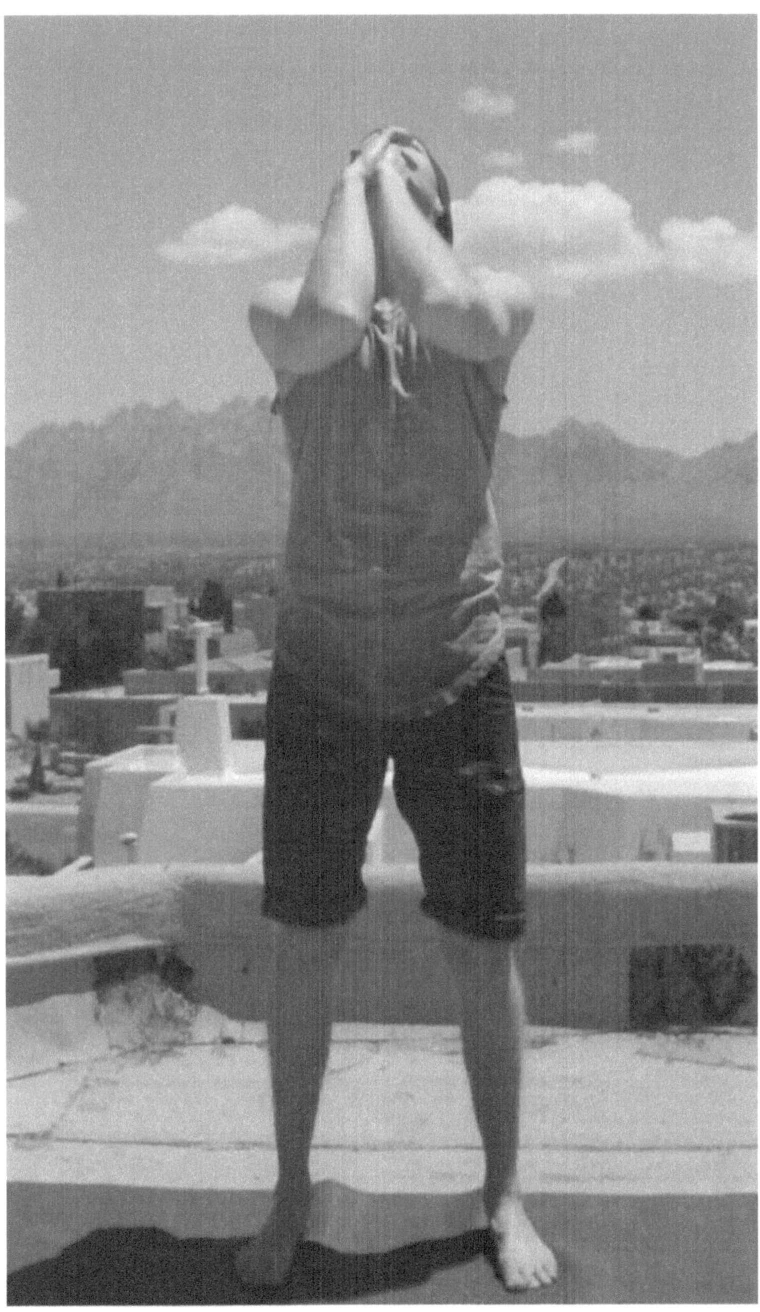

Please remember to keep your abdominal brace, and to maintain a neutral spine position. It can be tempting here to start leaning into a back bend, but I want you to keep your hips and spine locked in place the whole time. Keep

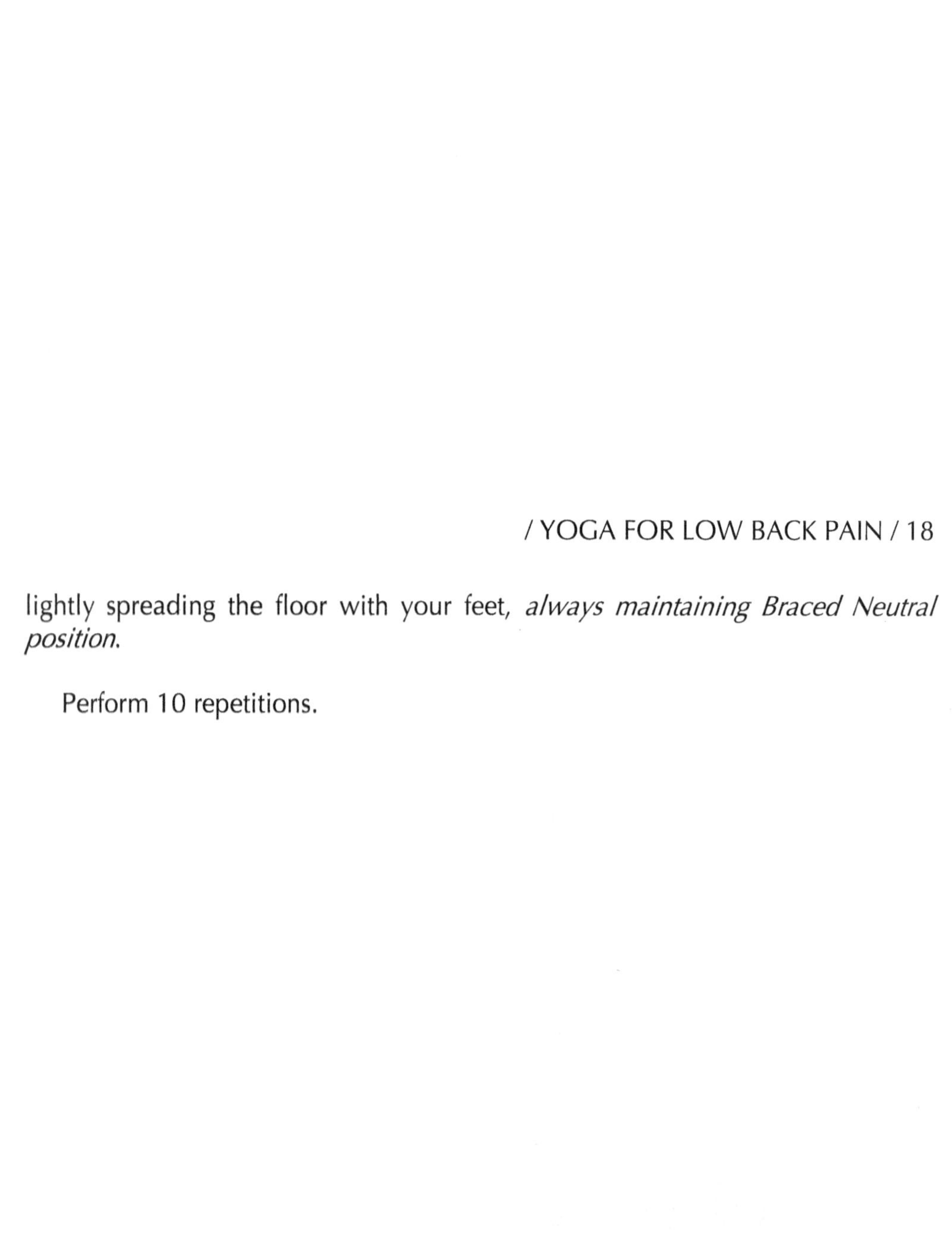

lightly spreading the floor with your feet, *always maintaining Braced Neutral position.*

Perform 10 repetitions.

CHAPTER FIVE

Spinal Elongation

1. Start in Braced Neutral Pose, then inhale deeply and raise your arms over your head, fingers *wide* open.

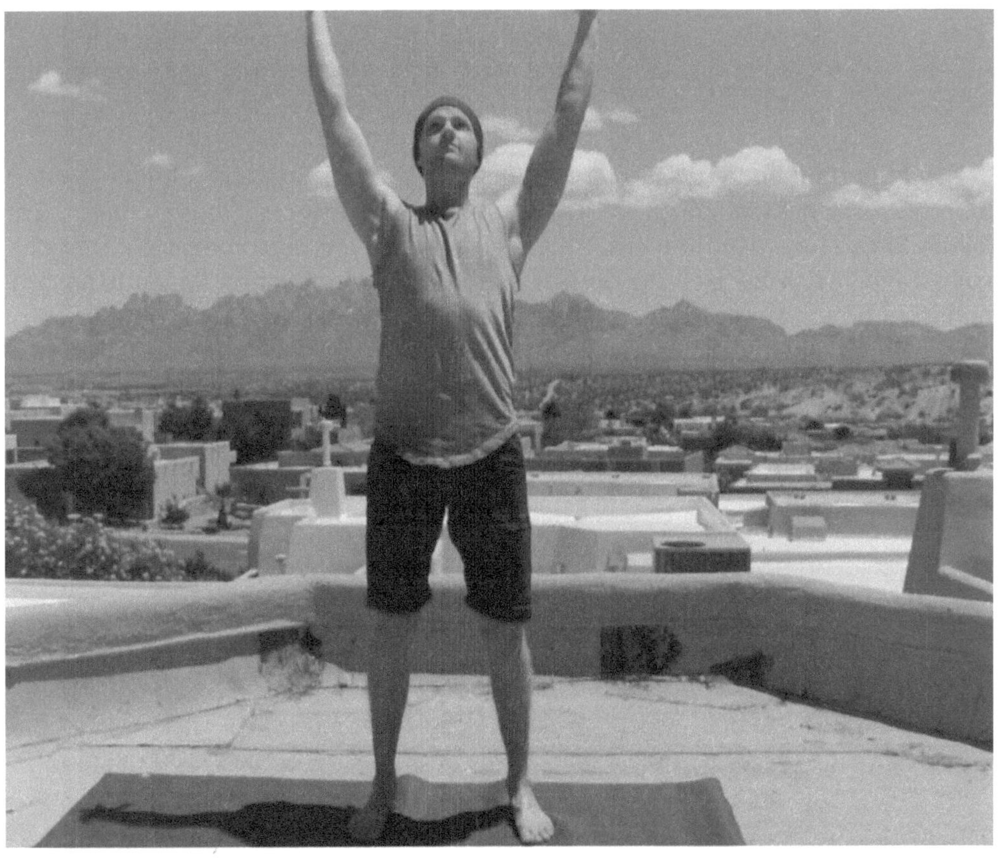

2. Now slide your shoulder blades down your back, pinching them slightly together, working at all times to maintain Braced Neutral Spine position. Really

squeeze your glutes, lightly pressing your hips forward into very *gentle* hip extension.

It's important not to go too far past neutral, so think less about bending *back* than about lengthening *up* through your chest, squeezing those glutes, and taking long, slow, deep breaths. This is a great decompression exercise for your spine, and it can be great to do this after you've been sitting for an extended period of time. Stay in this gentle back bend for three or four long, slow rounds of breathing, then exhale your arms back down to your sides, returning to Braced Neutral position.

CHAPTER SIX

Hip Hinge Progressions

PROGRESSION #1

1. Stand in Braced Neutral position, then inhale and hinge at the hips, leaning slightly forward and sliding your palms down along the sides of your quadriceps, until your palms reach your knees. Athletes will recognize this as essentially a deadlift movement pattern. Don't forget to maintain that 30%-ish contraction in your abs and obliques. Shoulders down and back, chest up.

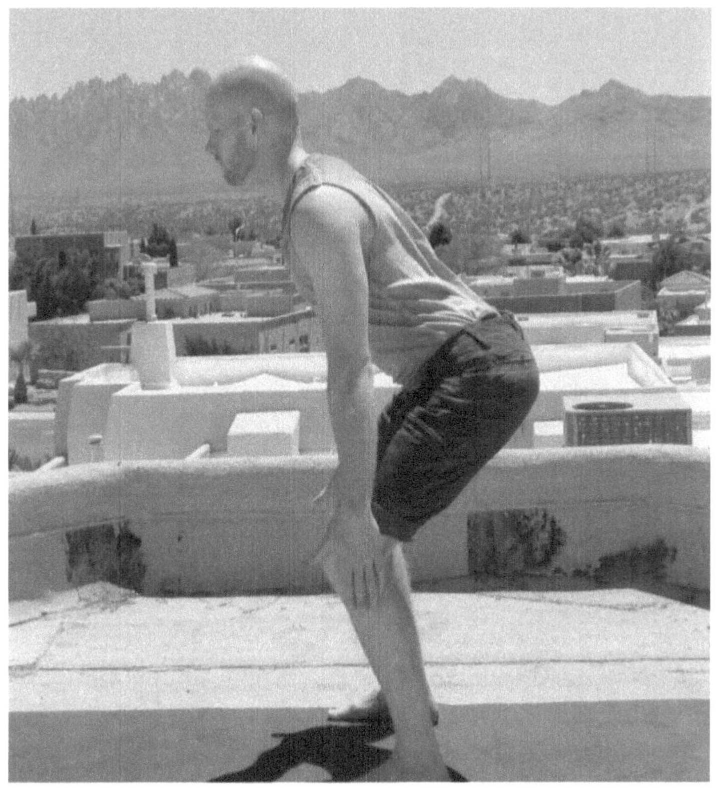

2. Pause for a moment at the bottom of the movement, then exhale and squeeze your glutes, pulling your hips through until you arrive back at the Braced Neutral standing position. Repeat 4 or 5 times.

PROGRESSION #2

1. This time I want you to take a long, slow inhale and extend your arms out to the sides, palms up.

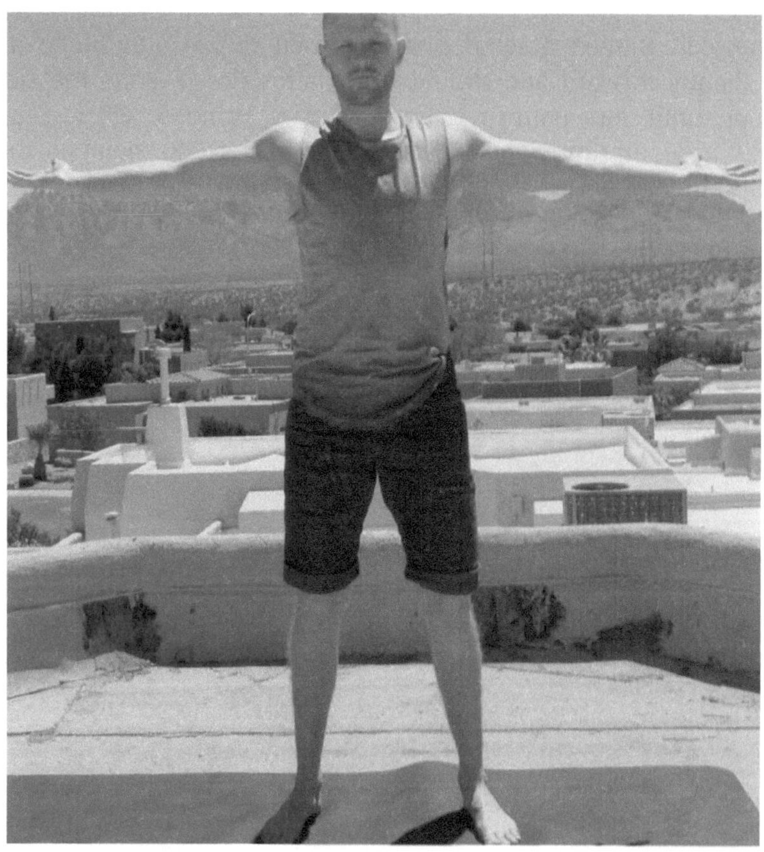

2. *Keep inhaling* as you hinge at the hips and bring your arms straight in front of you, rotating the palms down.

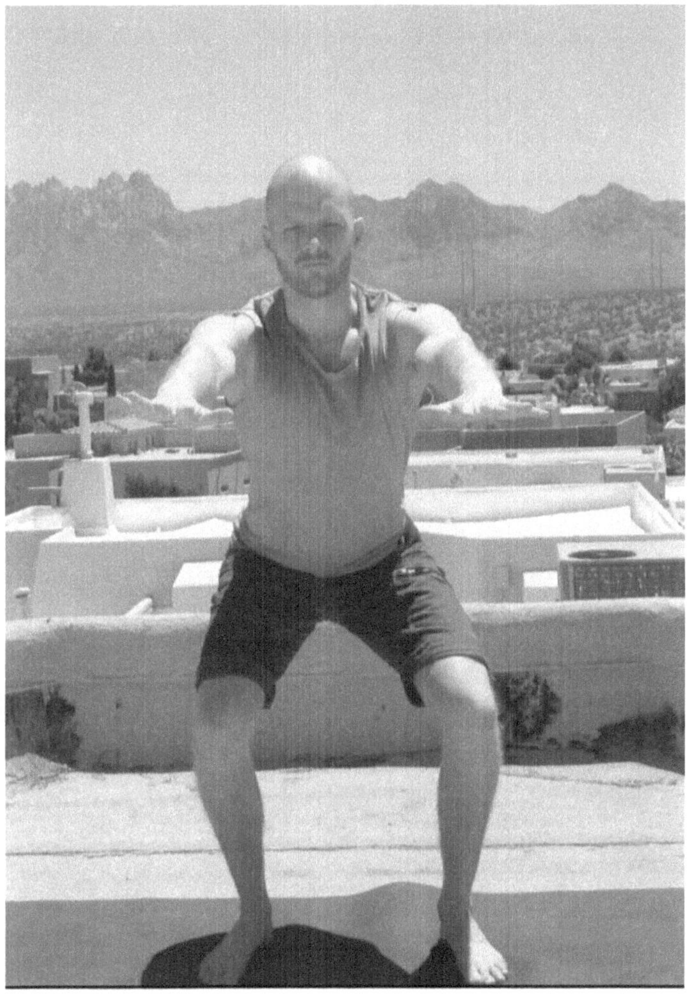

2. Pause at the bottom for a moment. Then *exhale* and squeeze your glutes to return to position 1. Repeat 4 or 5 times.

NOTE: For those of us with shear-intolerant backs (more on that later), this progression can be provocative to our pain, and should be skipped if it makes you feel worse.

PROGRESSION #3
1. Widen your stance and turn your toes out slightly. Now it's time for the *squat* progression. Everyone's comfortable squat stance is going to be different, so feel free to play around with it. I like to plant my feet pretty wide apart, much wider than hip's width, so it's almost a sumo-style squat stance.

2. Inhale your arms out and up over your head, slide your shoulders down, maintaining your abdominal brace, then sit straight down as low as you can

comfortably go. Keep your knees tracking over your middle toes, don't let them collapse inward!

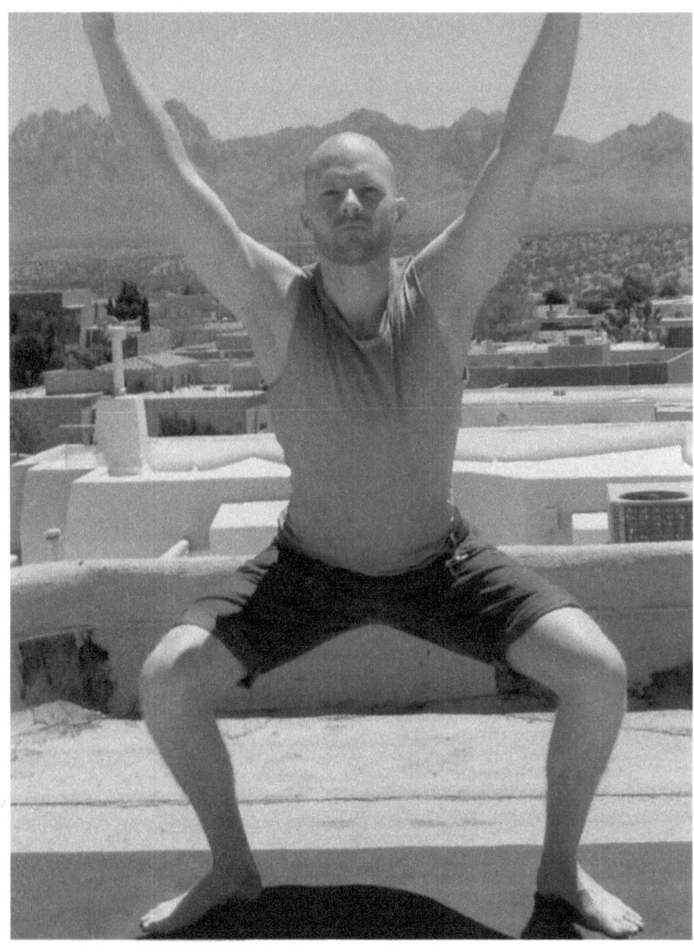

2. Pause at the bottom, then exhale and squeeze your glutes to return to a standing position, keeping your arms overhead. Repeat 4 or 5 times.

The preceding photo shows me at the absolute bottom of my safe squat depth, so as you can clearly see, I am not a naturally deep squatter! Like, at all. If you go so deep that your low back begins to collapse into flexion—trainers call this phenomenon the 'butt-wink'—then you'll cause far more problems than you solve. It's vital to maintain a perfectly braced, neutral and pain-free spine position. If you feel your lower back starting to round, or if you get even the *slightest* twinge of discomfort, don't be shy about squatting more shallowly.

Getting hung up on squat depth is dangerous and destructive if it causes you to break form and provokes your pain.

PROGRESSION #4

1. This final progression is the Deep Squat. In order to do a deep squat and maintain a neutral spine, I have to come all the way up on my tippytoes, like so:

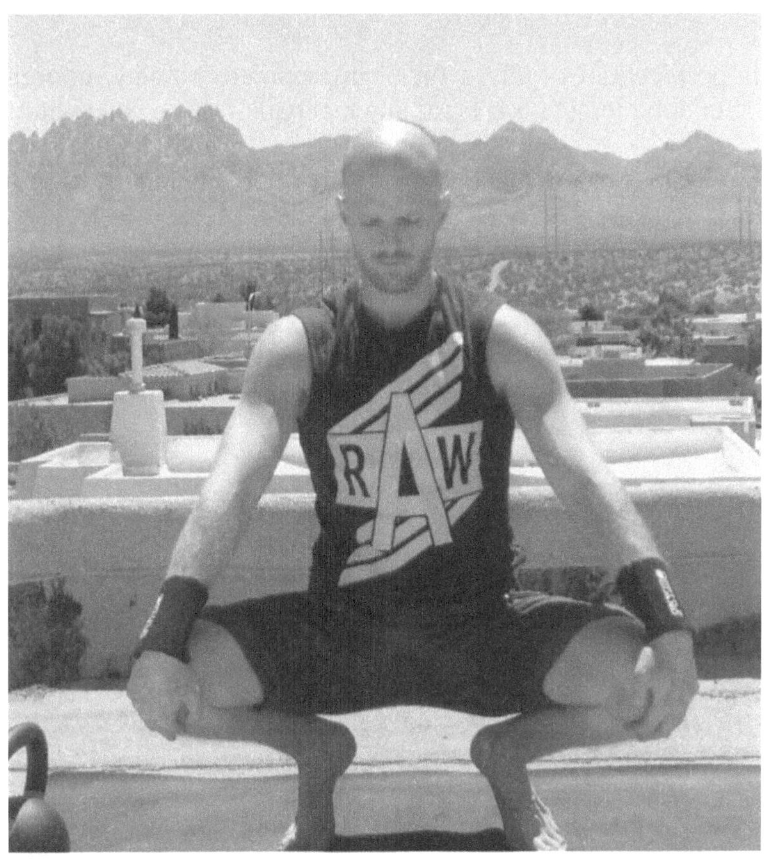

2. Go all the way down and touch your fingertips to the floor, without allowing your spine to 'break' into a rounded position. Hold here for a breath or two before coming back up. Obviously, if the knees complain at all, skip this variation for now.

CHAPTER SEVEN

Eagle

This pose requires quite a bit of appropriate mobility, coordination and balance, but don't forget good breathing mechanics while you're at it!

1. Start from Braced Neutral pose, then, on an inhale, raise your arms overhead.

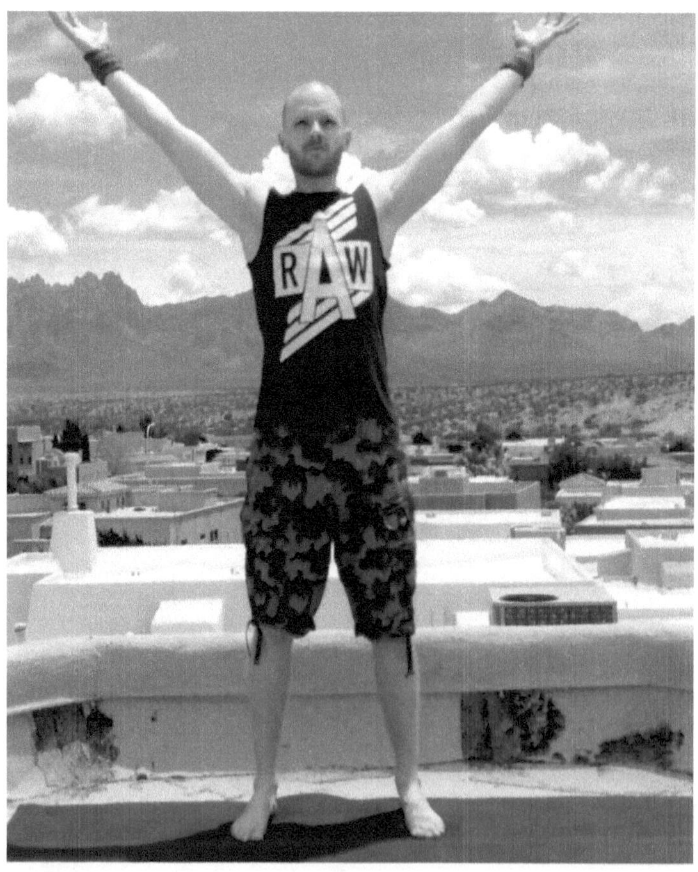

2. On the exhale, hook your right elbow under your left elbow, thumbs towards your face.

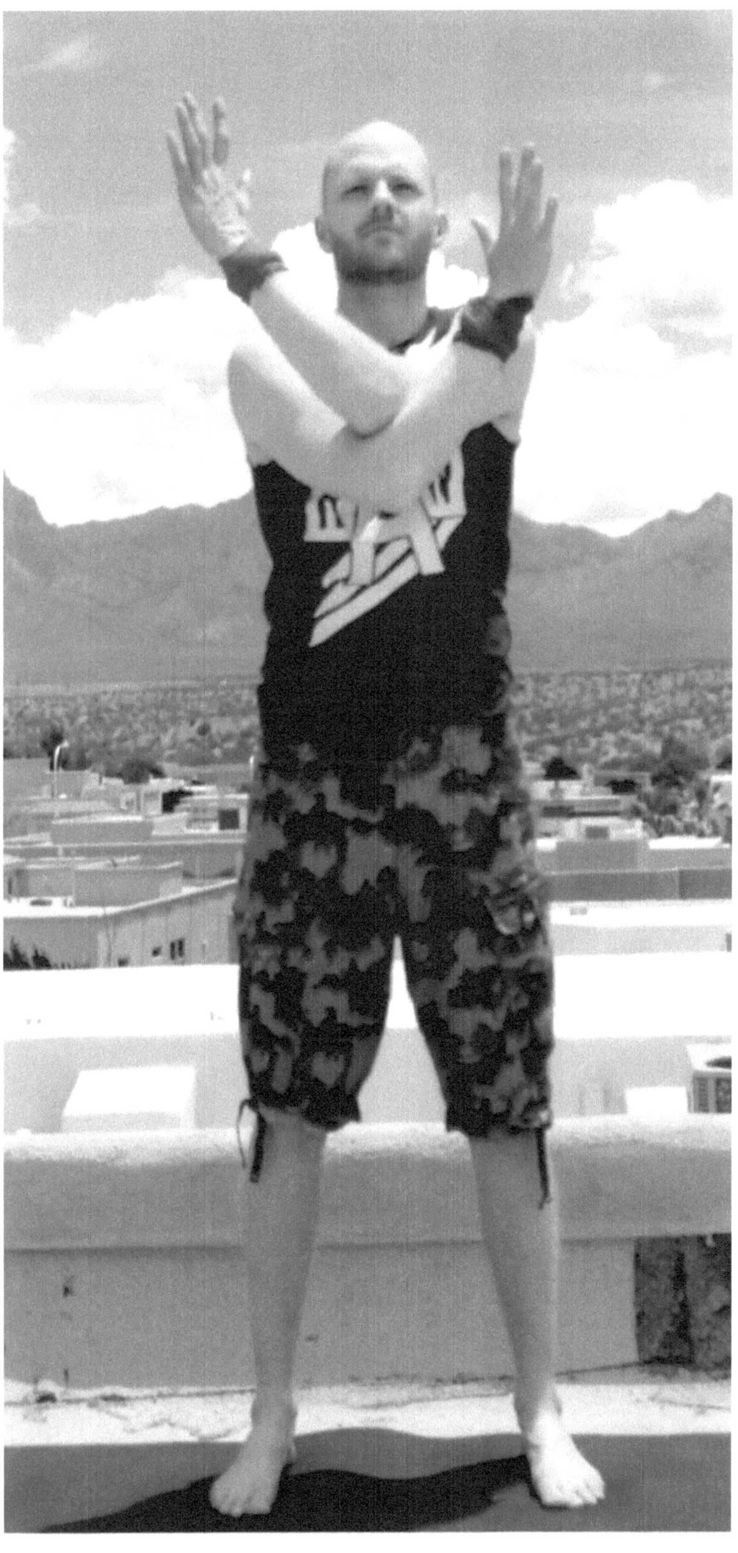

3. Here's where it gets tricky: Keeping your thumbs towards your face, take the long way round and grab your left thumb with your right fingertips.

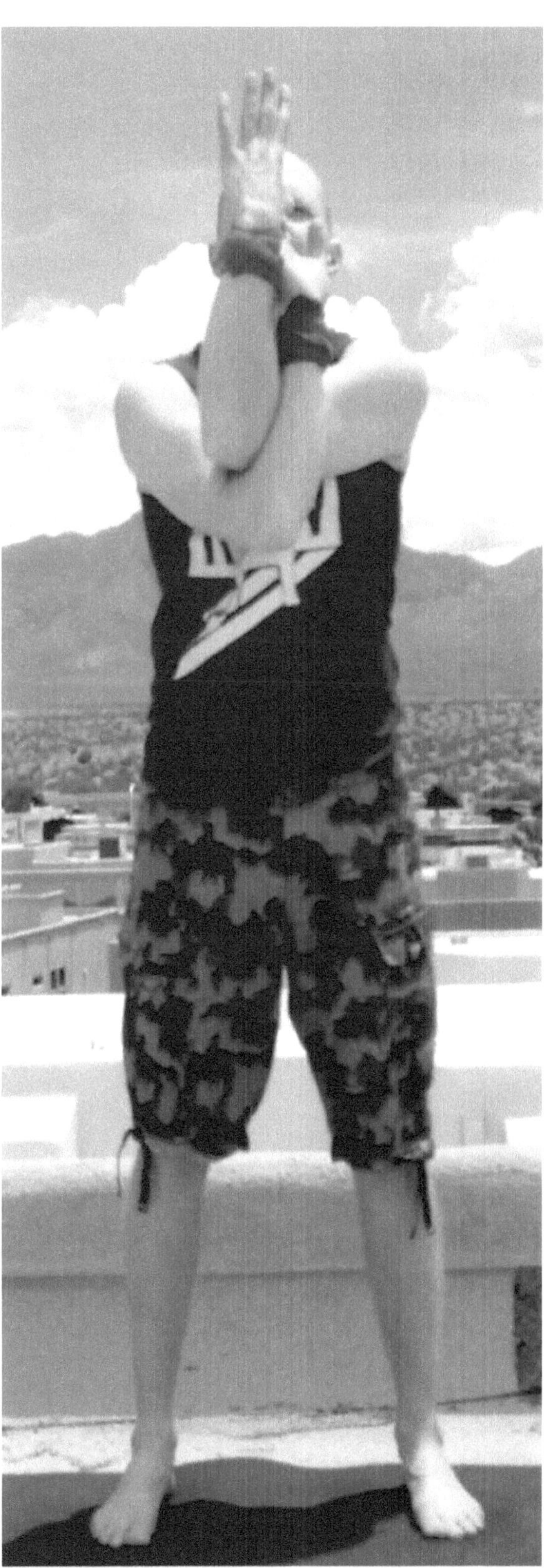

Alternatively, if your arms won't cooperate, simply grab your opposite shoulders, like so:

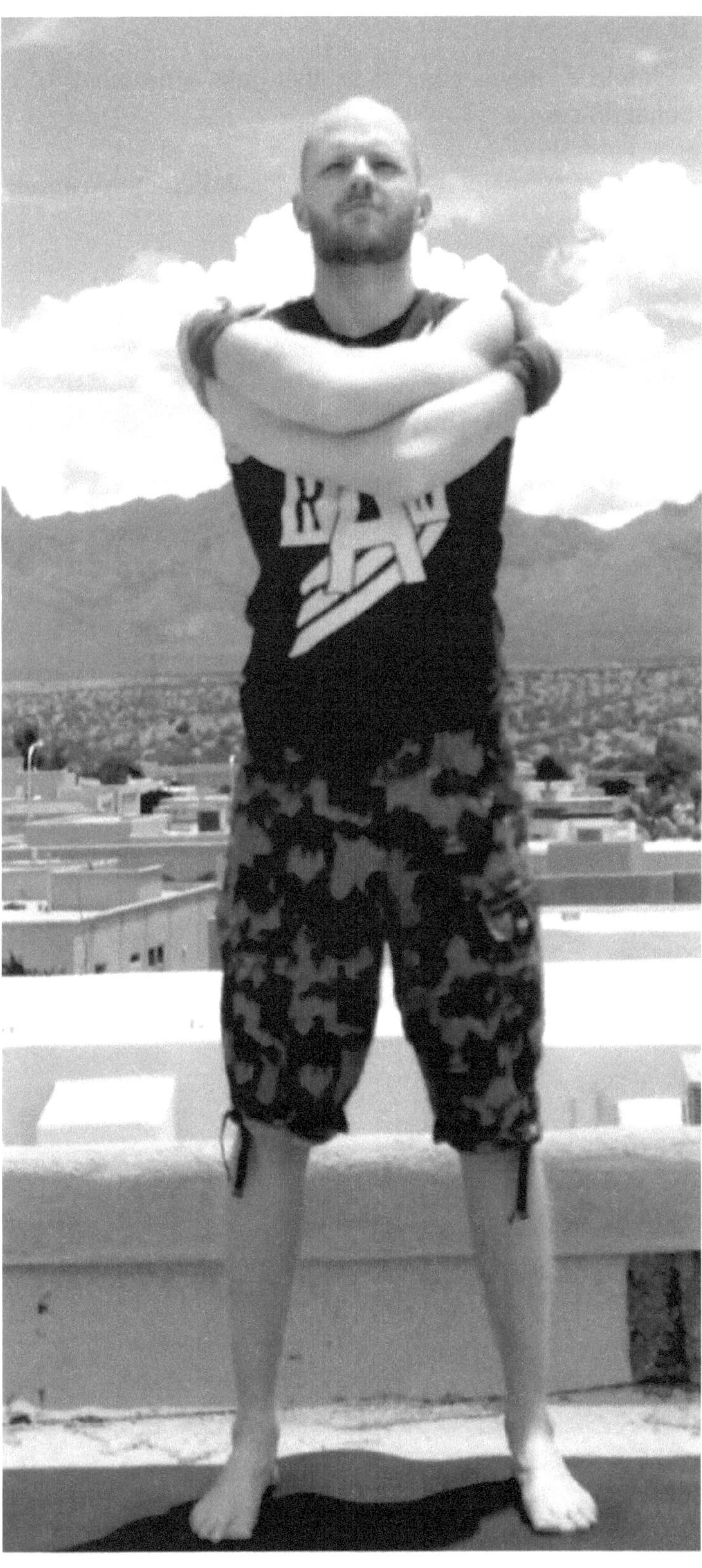

4. Slide your shoulders down your back, then take a moment to reconnect with your abdominal brace.

5. Now hinge at the hips, maintaining Braced Neutral Spine position.

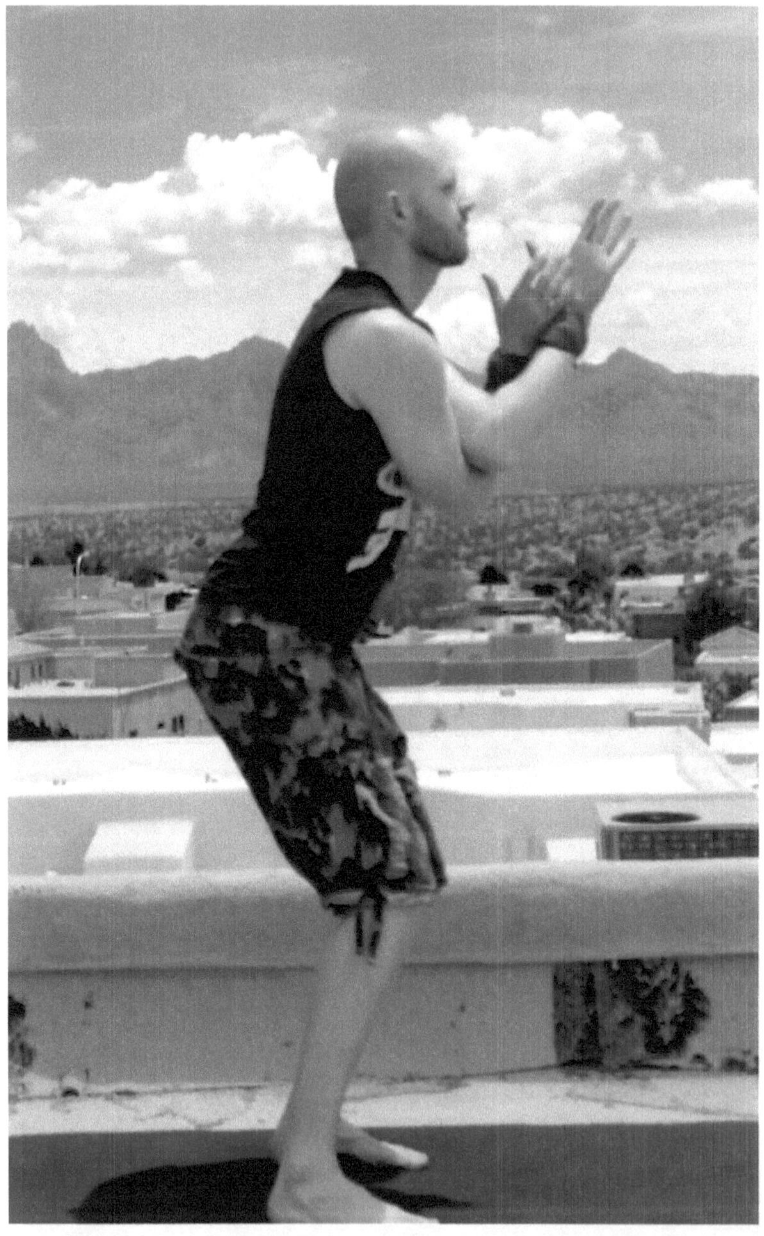

6. Finally, swing your right leg up and over your left leg. If possible, hook your right foot *behind* the left calf muscle.

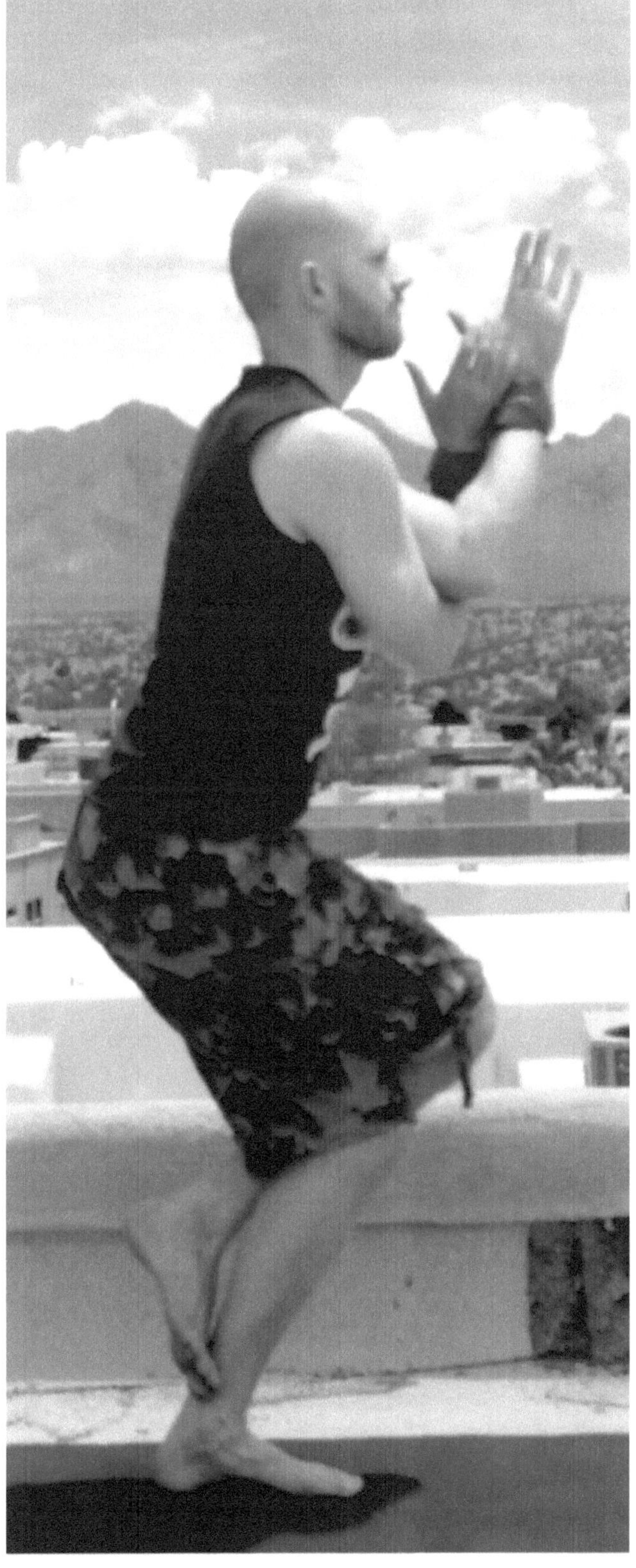

7. Continue to pull your elbows down but keep your chest up and your spine straight as you sit down, sinking as low as you go while maintaining your balance.

8. Find your safe maximum depth in the posture then hold the position for several rounds of calm, slow breathing through the nose.

9. Finally, on an inhale, un-pretzel yourself and return to Step 1, arms overhead, then repeat the same maneuver on the other side; this time swinging the left elbow under the right elbow. The left leg goes up and over the right leg.

10. Perform one to three rounds, depending on how well you can balance on one leg. If you find the balance too difficult for now, move on to Hip Airplane. You might find it more comfortable to practice your balance in that pose instead.

CHAPTER EIGHT

Hip Airplane

1. Starting from Braced Neutral position, inhale your arms out to the sides, like airplane wings, then step your right foot forward, bending slightly at the knee, and 'hinging' down from your right hip.

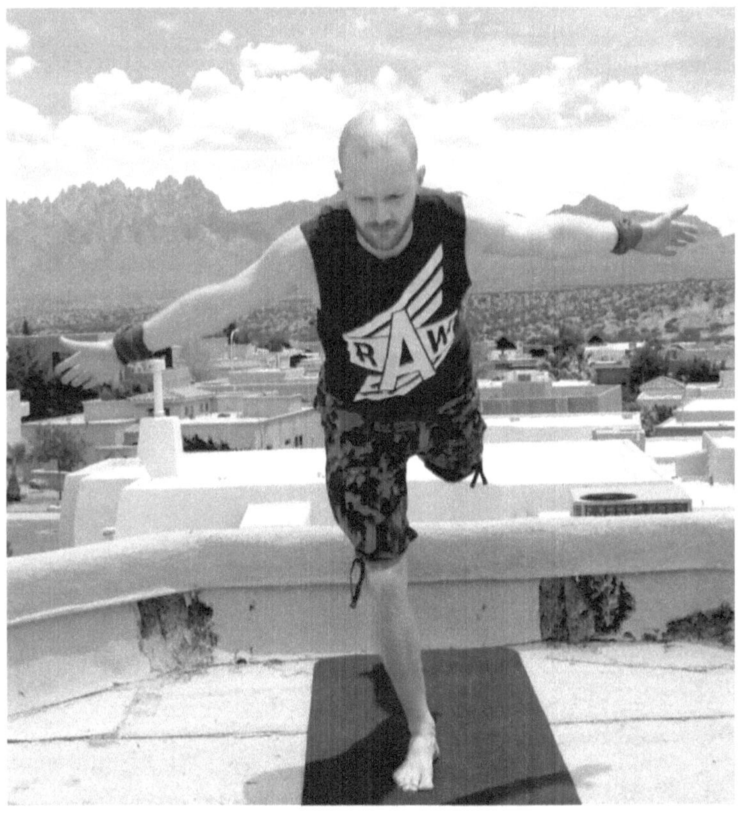

2. As you hinge down, make sure you maintain an even distribution of body weight on your right foot, keep your core tightly braced, and make sure your left glutes are engaged to keep your left leg lifted. The left leg should also be bended slightly at the knee, no need to keep it straight.

3. Once you've hinged down as far as you can *comfortably* go, reconnect to Braced Neutral then *slowly* rotate your left hip upward, letting your whole upper torso travel with you. Keep thinking about an even weight distribution on that right foot, because maintaining that is going to become much more tricky as you begin to rotate your hips.

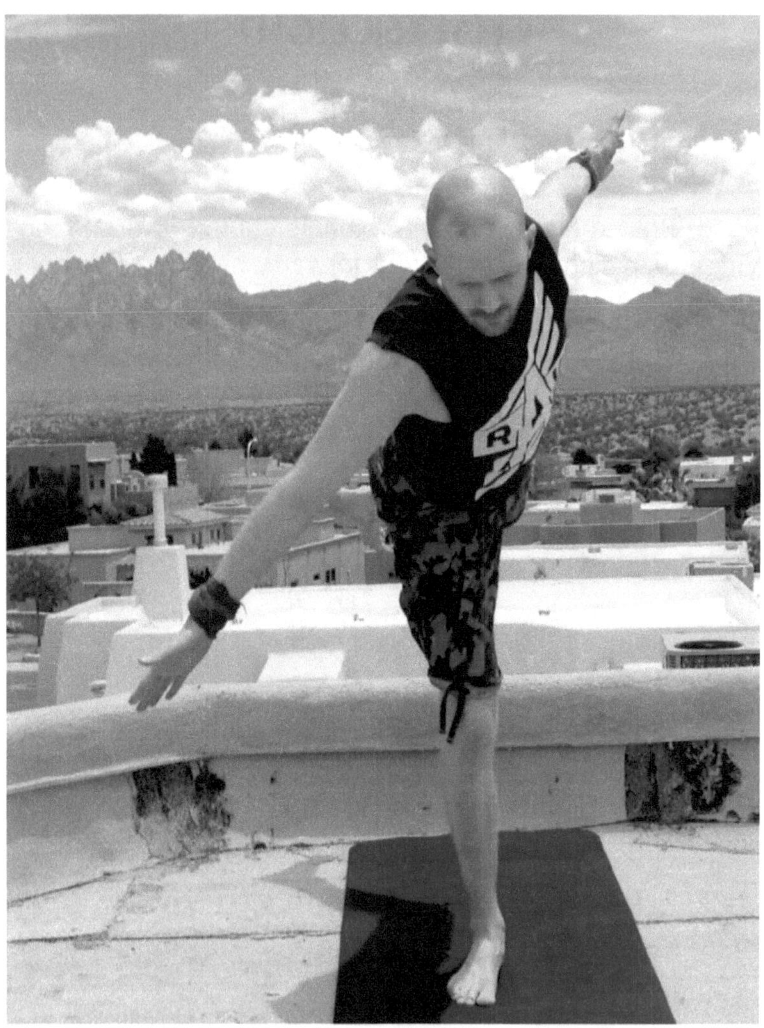

4. Pause for a moment at the top of your hip rotation—always breathing as calmly and slowly as possible through your nose, and making sure that your chest stays lifted—then rotate your hip back down.

5. Go for two or, at most, three hip rotations before stepping back into Braced Neutral Pose and then switching legs. This is a *very* challenging and fatiguing exercise, and if you overdo it you'll get into diminishing returns territory pretty quickly. Due to the nature of this posture, fatigue and poor form

can easily cause those pesky micro-movements of the spinal joints that can provoke pain, so less is more.

CHAPTER NINE

Triangle 1

1. Begin by standing in Braced Neutral position, with your palms in prayer position in front of your chest. Then take a wide step to the side with your right foot, bringing your arms straight out to the side, turning your right foot all the way to the right while keeping your left foot pointing straight ahead.

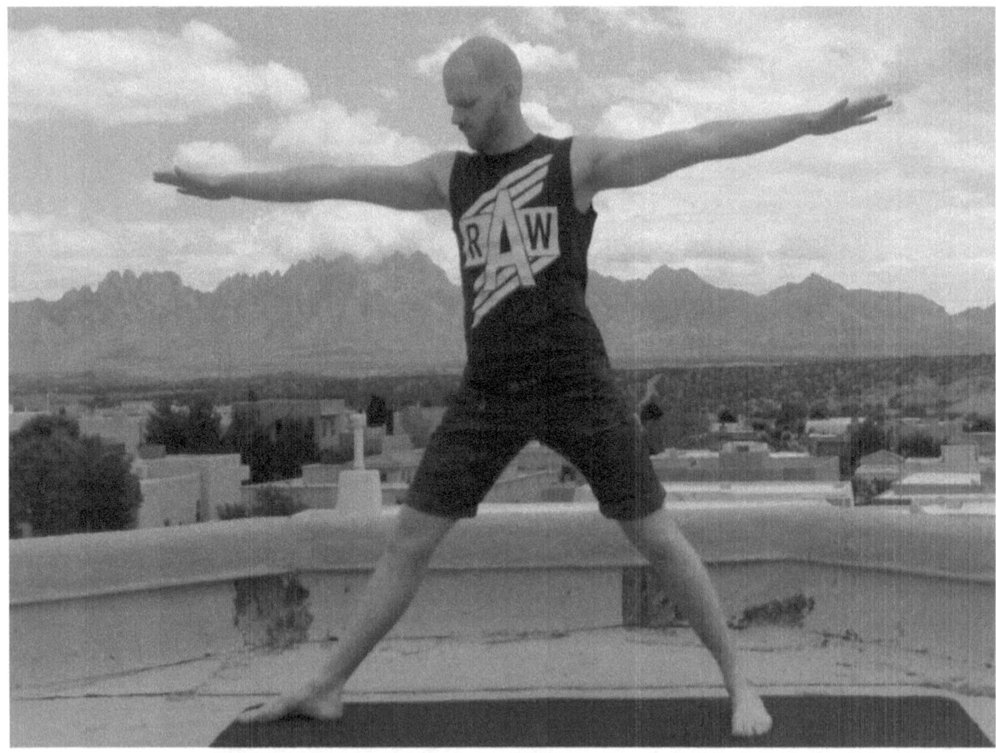

2. Keep your left leg straight, and really squeeze your right quads so that you're sure your right leg is completely straight. Maintain that contraction in your right quads as you windmill your arms straight up and down.

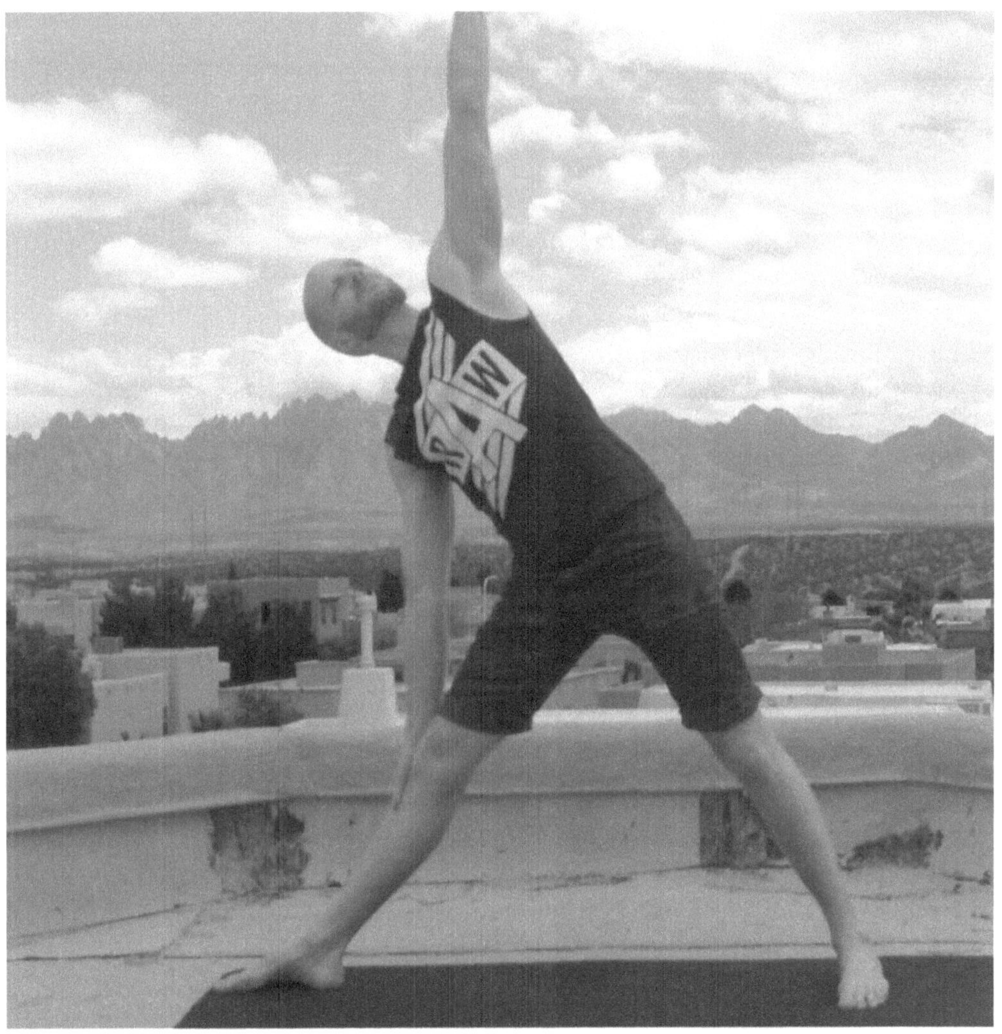

3. Make sure you continue to brace your spine with a gentle abdominal contraction, breathing calmly and slowly through your nose. Make certain that your right knee tracks over your middle toes, keep your shoulders down away from your ears, and maintain a straight line from your left hipbone all the way up to your left armpit; no rounding the spine! Practice in front of a mirror if you need to *see* it…sometimes the spine can begin to round here and it can be hard to *feel* it. This posture should create a gentle stretching sensation in your right hamstrings. Maintain for at two or three rounds of calm, slow breathing on each side.

CHAPTER TEN

Triangle 2

1. Take a slightly wider stance than you did for Triangle 1. Turn your right foot to the right, then bend your right knee, making sure not to let the knee collapse inward. (Aim the knee towards your middle toes.) The knee should be more or less directly above your ankle. Don't let the knee go beyond the ankle, and make sure to press through your right heel at all times. This will prevent you from just "sinking" into the posture and "hanging out." The left quad is engaged tightly to keep the left leg straight. The outside edge of the left foot should be pressing into the floor, don't let it roll up.

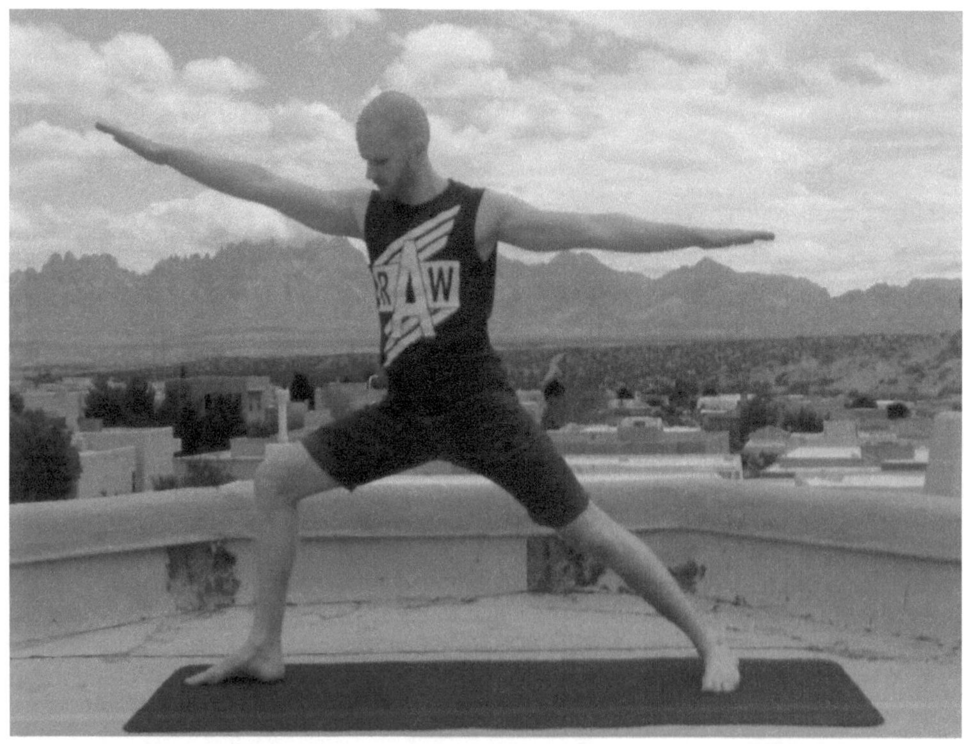

2. Windmill your arms. There is a tendency for the arms to want to collapse *inward*; don't let this happen, keep your chest open *wide*. Feel the opening sensation in your chest and even in the anterior deltoids. Keep your shoulders down away form your ears, and work to maintain an absolutely straight line from your left heel all the way up to your left armpit. Braced, neutral spine at all times. Breathe calmly and slowly through your nose for two or three rounds, then switch sides.

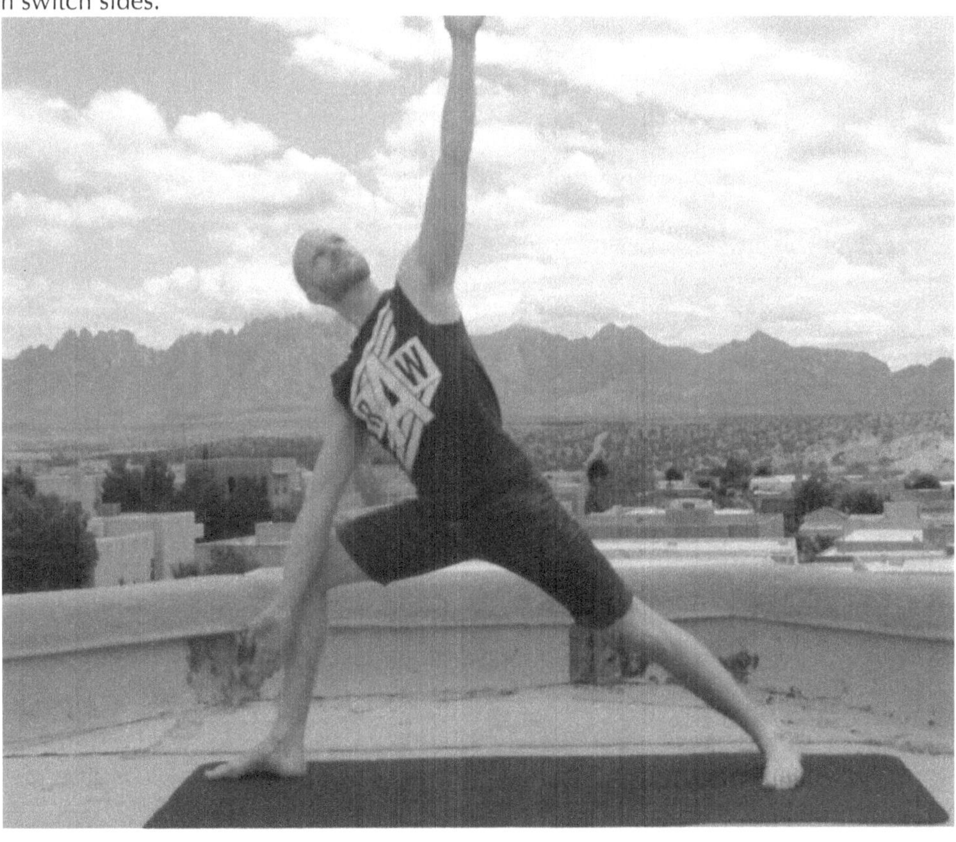

CHAPTER ELEVEN

Reverse Lunges

Forward lunges are fine, if you have bulletproof knees, but I always encourage my students to adopt the much more knee-friendly *reverse* lunge. In the forward lunge variation, the lengthening of the quadricep muscles under load can cause strain through the patella. Reverse lunges, however, do a better job of activating the posterior chain musculature and allow for a slightly higher hip flexion angle, the practical upshot of which is that the rectus femoris muscle can be more relaxed in that lengthening-under-load (*eccentric*) phase of the movement, causing less strain on the patella.

1. Stand at the top of your yoga mat and step back with your right foot, then go ahead and drop your right knee all the way to the ground. Your knee doesn't necessarily need to touch the ground when you're performing your repetitions, but here we're just working on the form.

NOTE: the back foot is always dorsiflexed (toes tucked under), which might cause issues if you suffer from plantar fasciitis, posterior tibial tendinitis, or other types of foot pain. As always, if any posture exacerbates existing symptoms—not *just* your back pain—leave it alone for now!

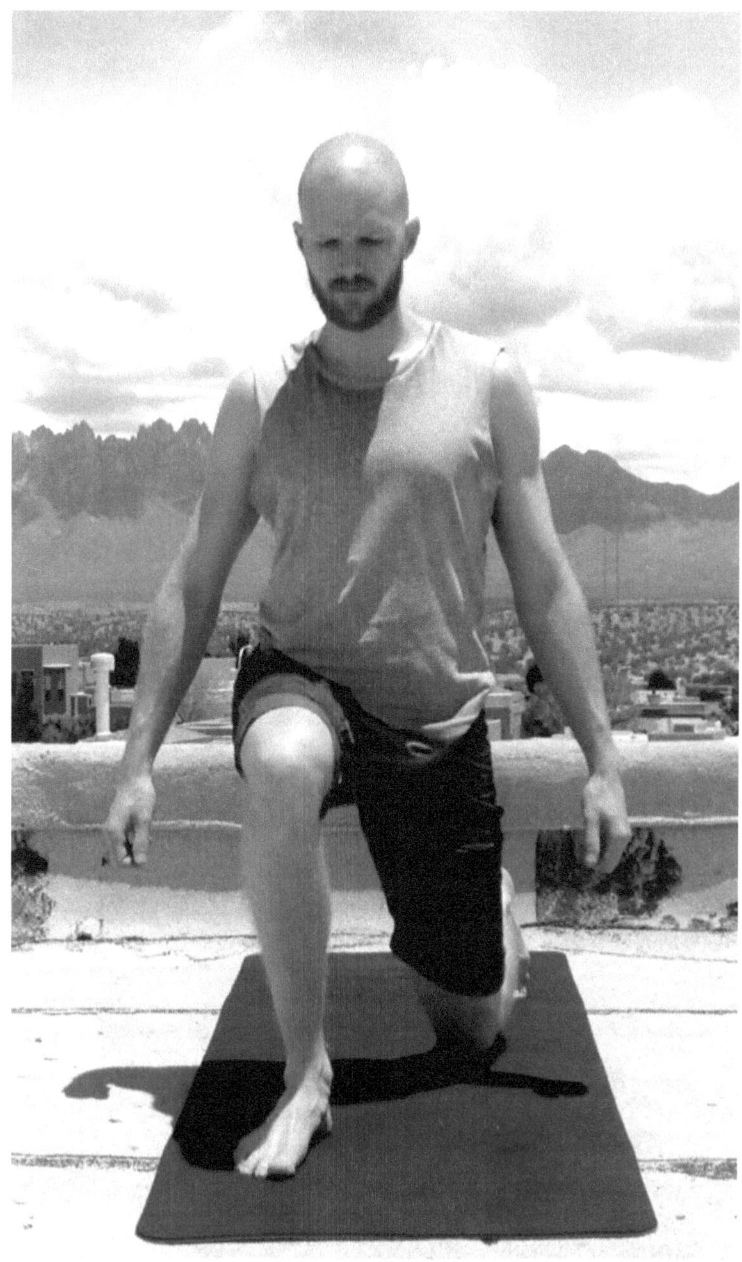

2. You'll probably notice that whatever leg is forward, that hip wants to hike heavenward, as in the picture below. For our purposes, always focusing on good spinal alignment, this is obviously sub-optimal, so see if you can sink that hip down a bit so that both hips and shoulders are more-or-less in good alignment.

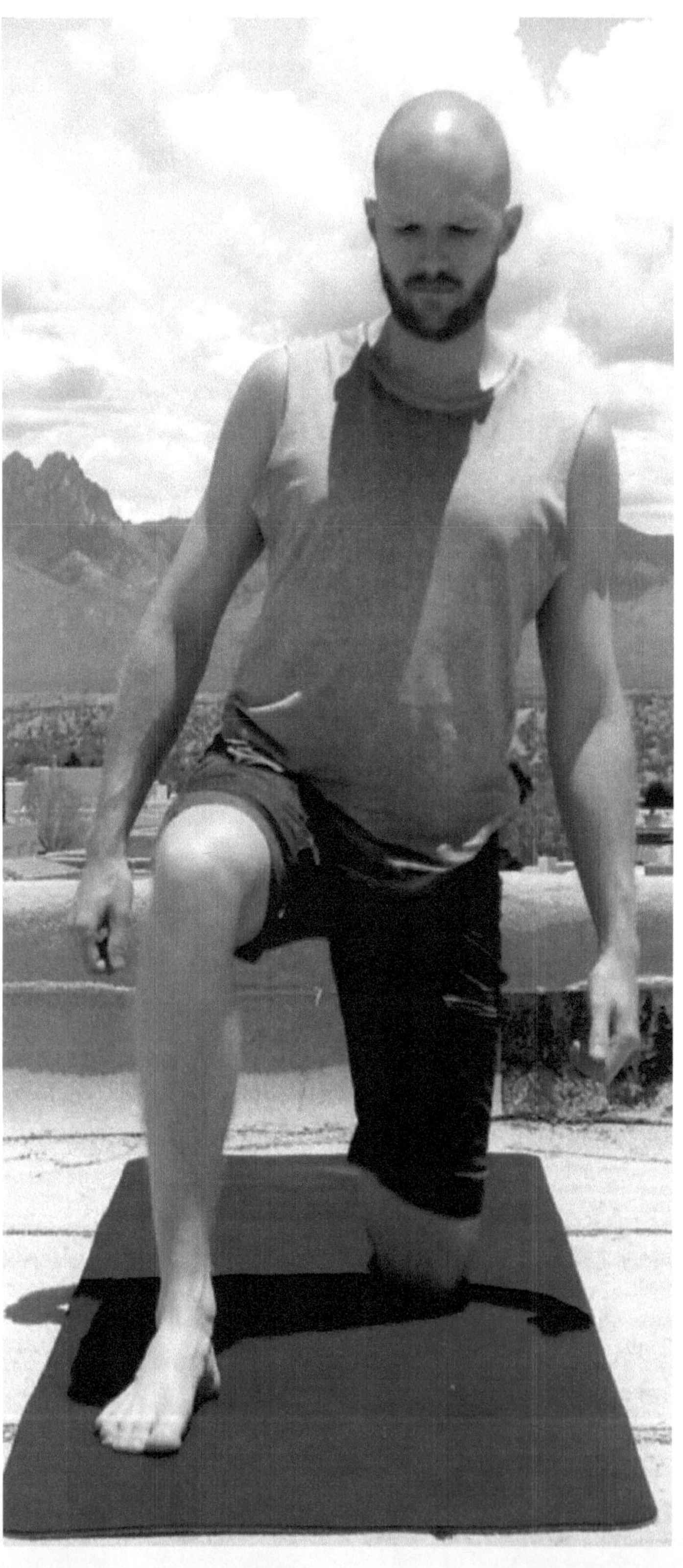

3. Once you've leveled off your hips, notice the position of the back hip in relation to the front knee. I usually find that the back hip wants to be *too far* back, and that the front knee wants to collapse outward, like so:

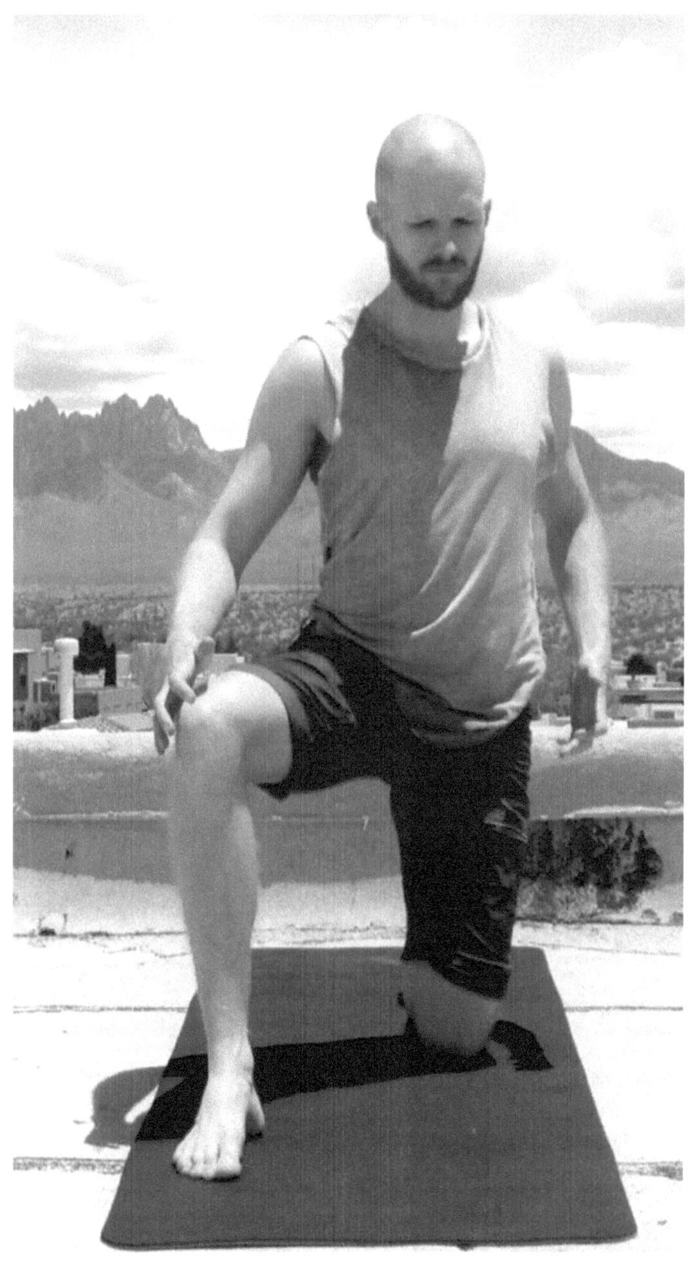

4. Just imagine there are little magnets pulling your left hip and the inside of your right knee slightly *toward* one another. Also, the front knee is tracking towards the middle toes, rather than collapsing in or winging out.

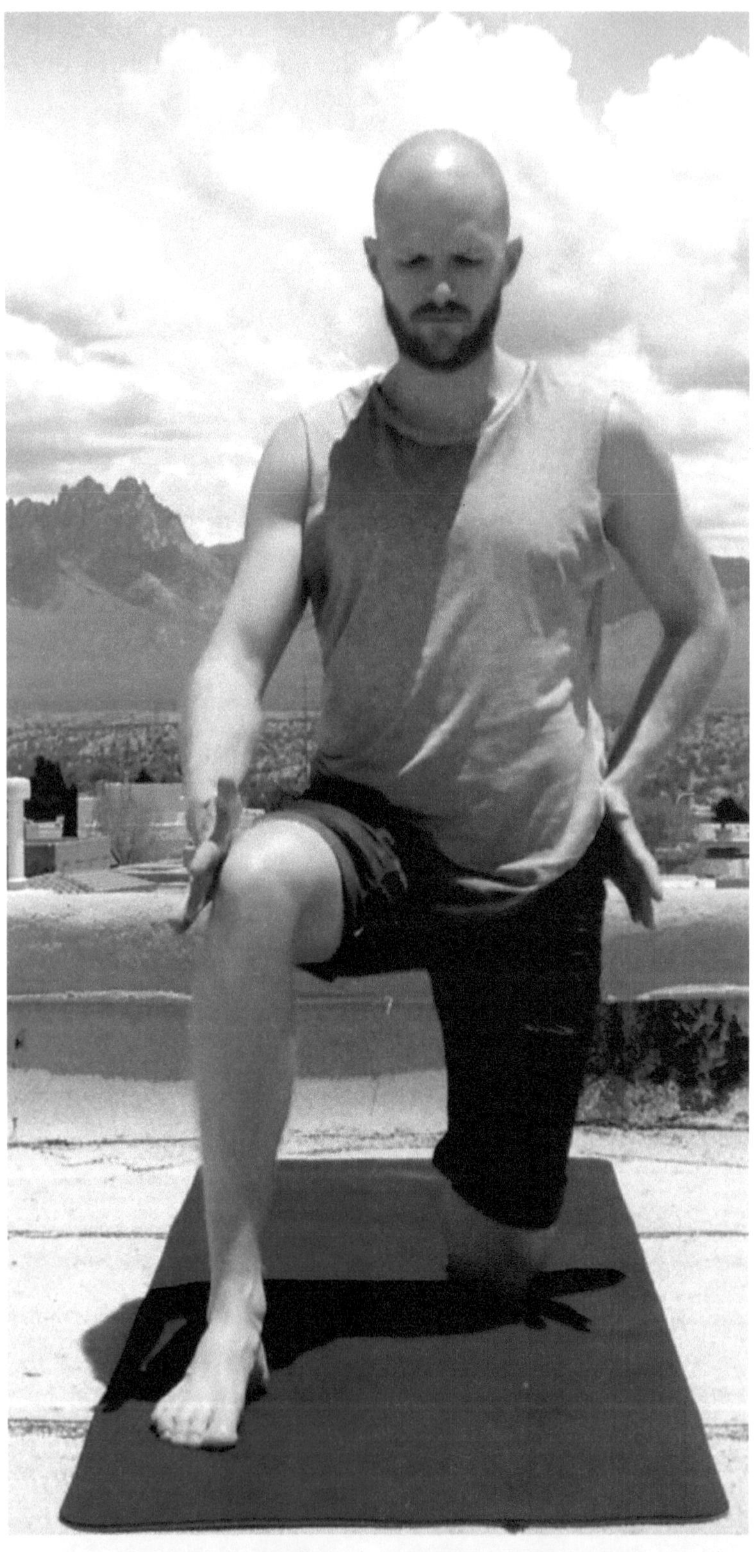

5. The last step is to raise your left arm up over your head. This really helps to open up the whole front side of your body, and if your hip flexors are chronically short and tight—and chances are, that's the case—don't be surprised if you start to *really* feel the stretch in the left hip flexor as soon as you raise that arm overhead.

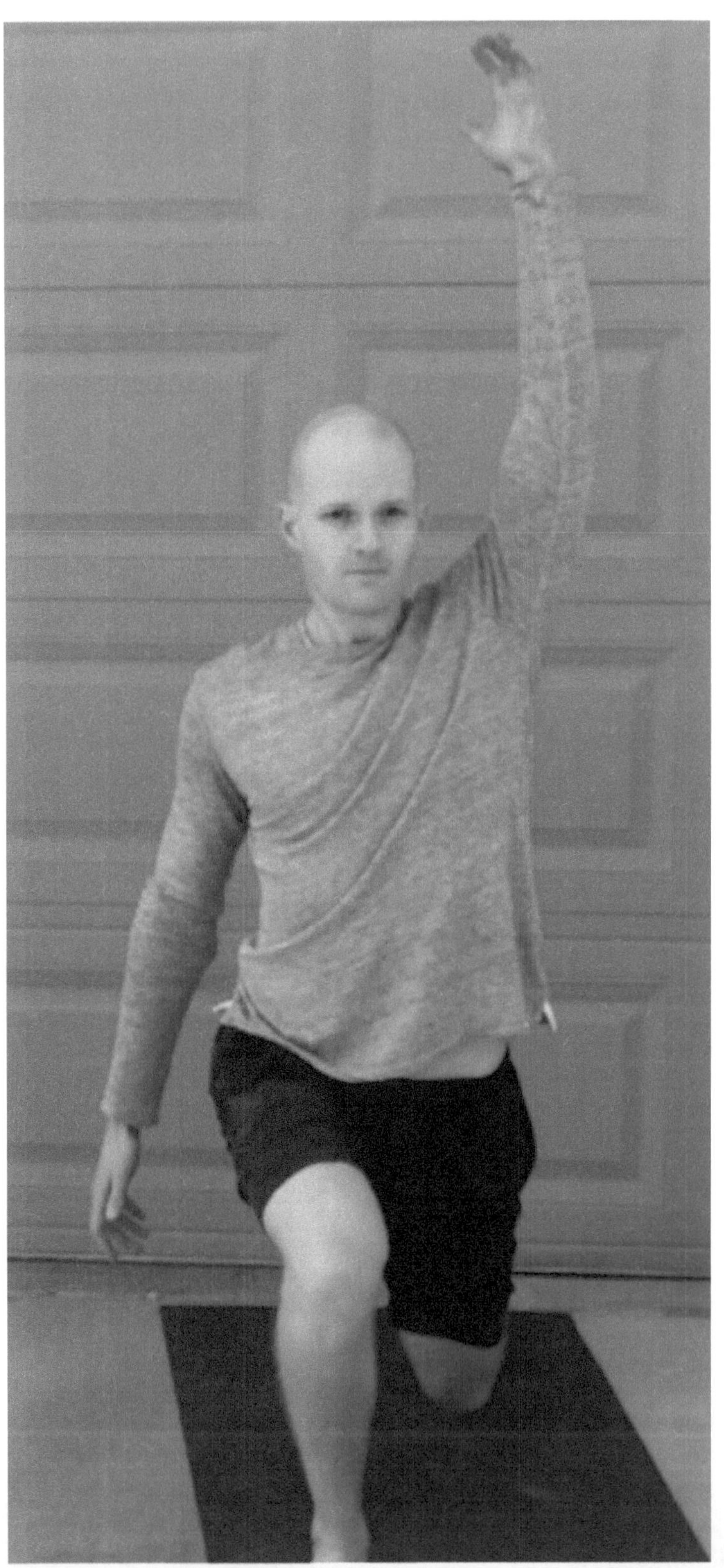

6. So that's the basic body position you want to achieve when you step backward into your lunge. When stepping forward again to the top of your yoga mat, work on pressing down through your right *heel* to come up, returning to Braced Neutral Pose before stepping back with the oppose leg.

Perform 8 reverse lunges on each leg. Start with one set, progressing to 2 or 3 sets, but don't be in a hurry to do multiple sets. This is really complex movement that requires a tremendous amount of balance and patience to execute with proper form.

Eventually, you can graduate to loading this movement with a kettlebell, either held by your side, pressed overhead, or held at your shoulder in the rack position. This is a great way to asymmetrically load the movement, encouraging strength and endurance:

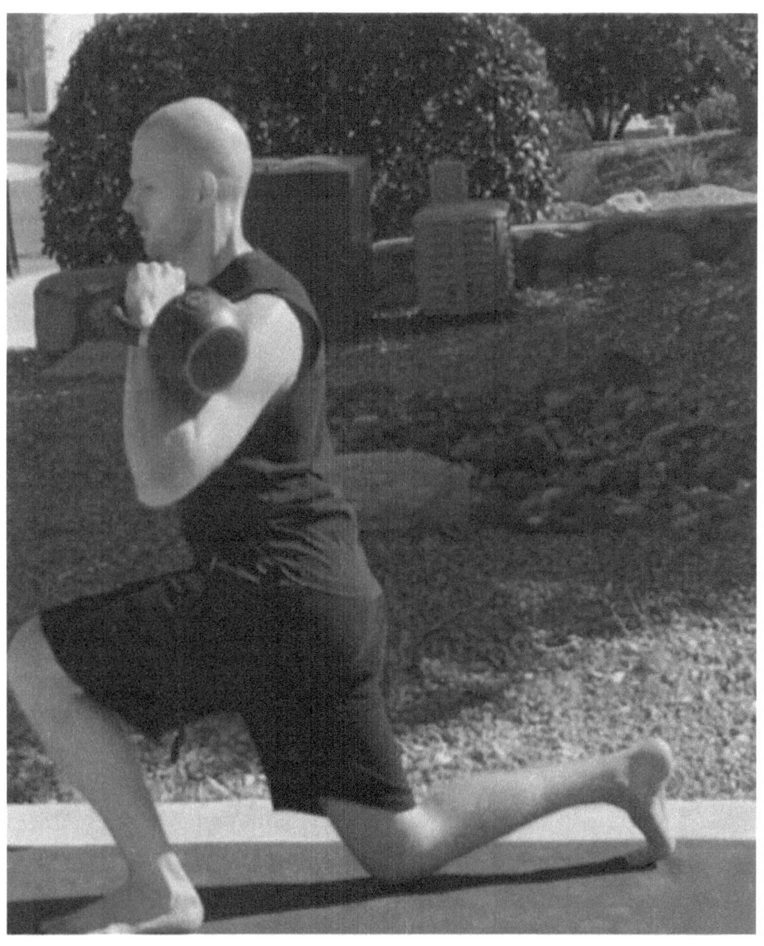

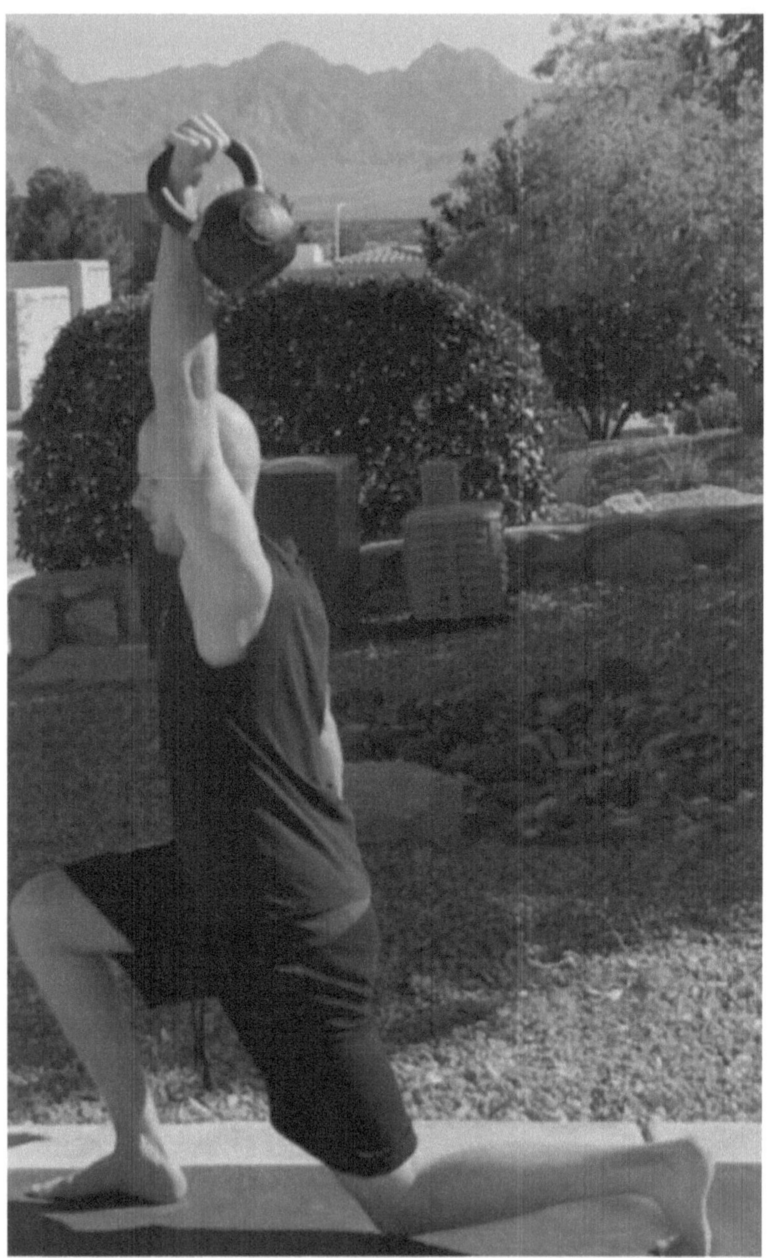

I have found this to be one of the very best movements for 'waking up' sleepy gluteal muscles and hamstrings. Since most of us with low back pain tend to be pretty weak in these posterior chain muscles, don't be surprised if even just one set of 8 bodyweight reverse lunges makes you feel sore the next day. But as long is it's not aggravating your pain, stick with it!

CHAPTER TWELVE

Belly-Down Corpse Pose

According to Dr. Stu McGill, writing in his book *Back Mechanic,* low back pain can produce "antalgia," which means a loss of the natural hollow in the lower spine; a "flattening" of the low back, in other words.

Belly Down Corpse Pose can help to restore that natural lordotic curve. Focus on really relaxing all your muscles when you're in this position:

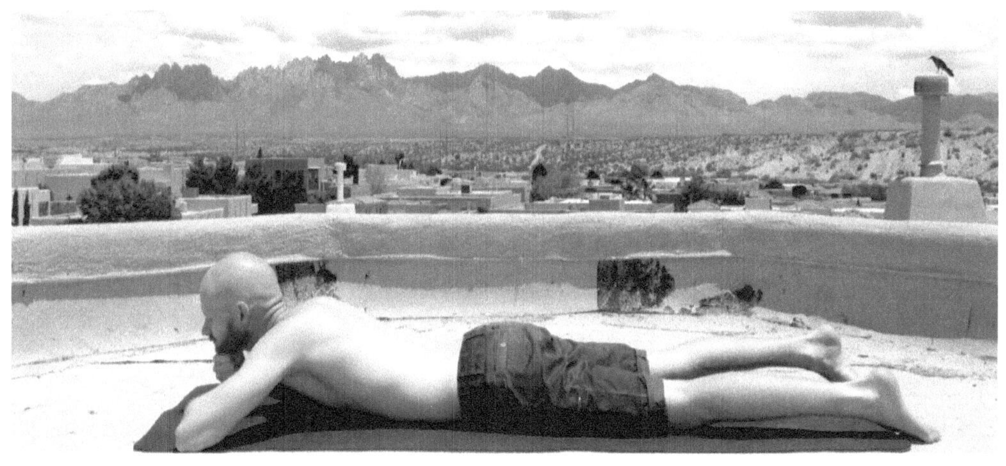

You can either rest your chin on your two fists, as Dr. McGill recommends and as I'm demonstrating here, or you can simply make a "pillow" with your palms and rest your forehead on top of them.

While in Belly Down Corpse Pose, take the opportunity to run a quick diagnostic on yourself. How do you feel? Is your pain level higher or lower than you started?

Hopefully, you feel at least a little bit better. If you don't, experiment with fewer exercises next time you practice the standing sequence. Chances are, one or more of these exercises are provocative to your specific pain. If you do feel better, however, congratulations! If you're accustomed to the type of yoga that beats the tar out of your body with excessive 'stretching' and spinal flexion, this will be a novel feeling.

Hang out here for 2 to 4 minutes, focusing on your calm and slow breathing, before moving on to the floor sequence.

CHAPTER THIRTEEN

Cat-Camel

This is the posture I'm sure a lot of yogis have been waiting for, those of you with prior yoga experience who *still* crave some movement in the spine despite all this talk about bracing and strengthening and locking the spine into a pain-free position and not letting it move.

Dr. Stu McGill, in his laboratory studies, found that the least stressful way to achieve spinal motion is via the Cat-Camel pose. However, in *The Back Mechanic*, Dr. McGill stresses that the goal is *not* to "stretch," and that pushing this posture into the every end-range of your motion is **not** a good idea; he goes so far as to suggest that practitioners slightly *reduce* their range of motion so they're not reaching the extreme in either the cat or the camel phases.

1. From belly-down corpse pose, brace your spine and carefully transition onto all fours. Then, for Cat, inhale and raise your head and your tailbone towards the sky, whilst letting your midsection "sag" towards the floor. This is one of the few times in the sequence where I will discourage you from "bracing" your spine; on the contrary, I want you keep your core totally relaxed. The inhaling Cat phase should be held for about four seconds.

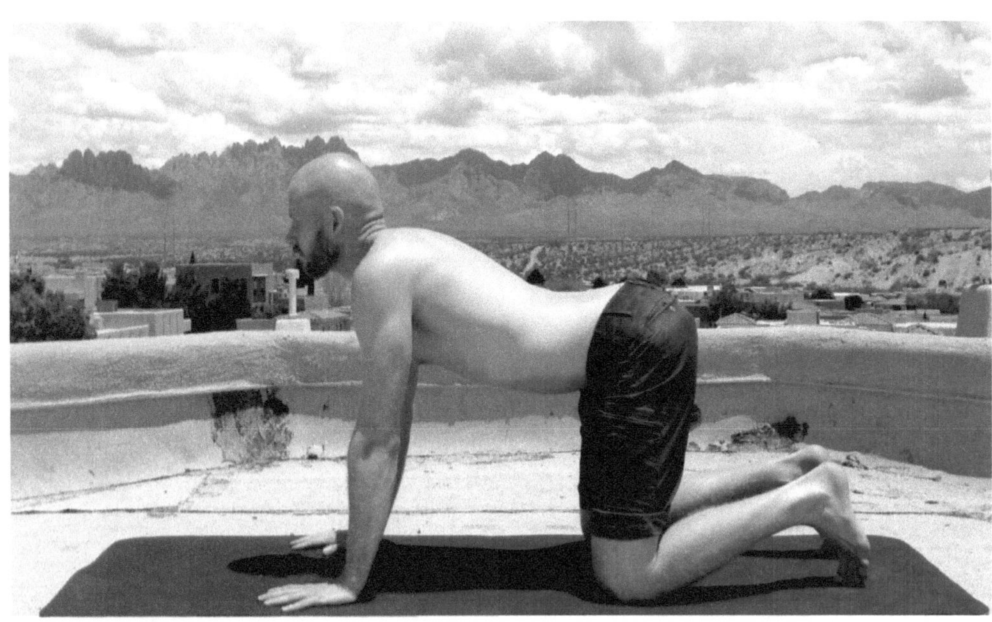

2. To transition into the Camel phase, slowly exhale (also for a four second count) and tuck your chin to your chest whilst tucking your tailbone under.

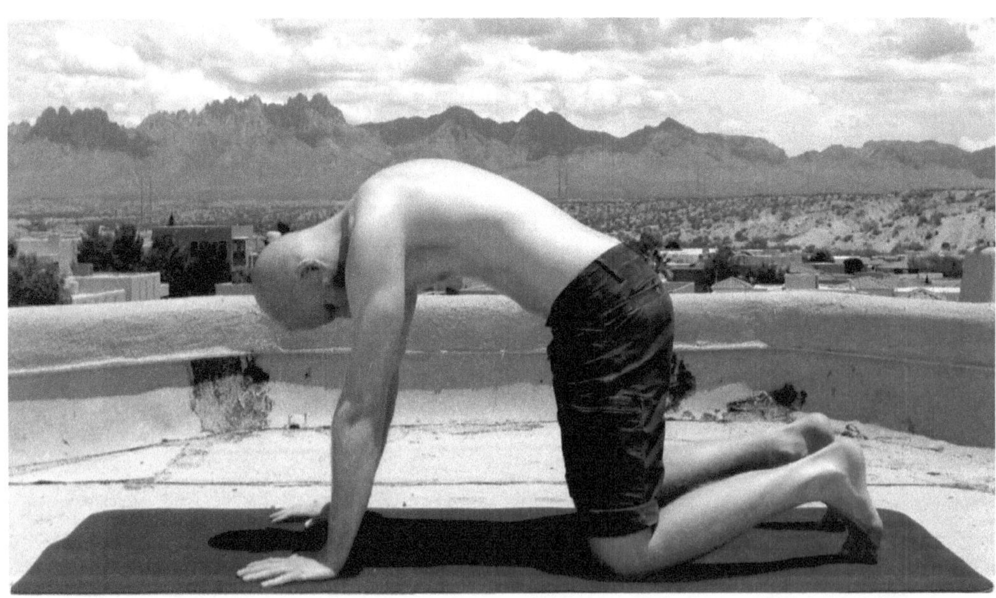

Seven to eight repetitions were found to be optimal for reducing spine friction and resistance to motion, whereas further repetitions were found to be counter-productive.

CHAPTER FOURTEEN

Bird Dog

This simple movement is a great exercise for your back extensors.

1. Start on all fours, locking your spine into a braced neutral position. No rounding or collapsing backs. Nice, tight abdominal contraction. Think about spreading the floor apart with your palms to lock your shoulders into position as well.

2. Lift your right leg and left arm up simultaneously.

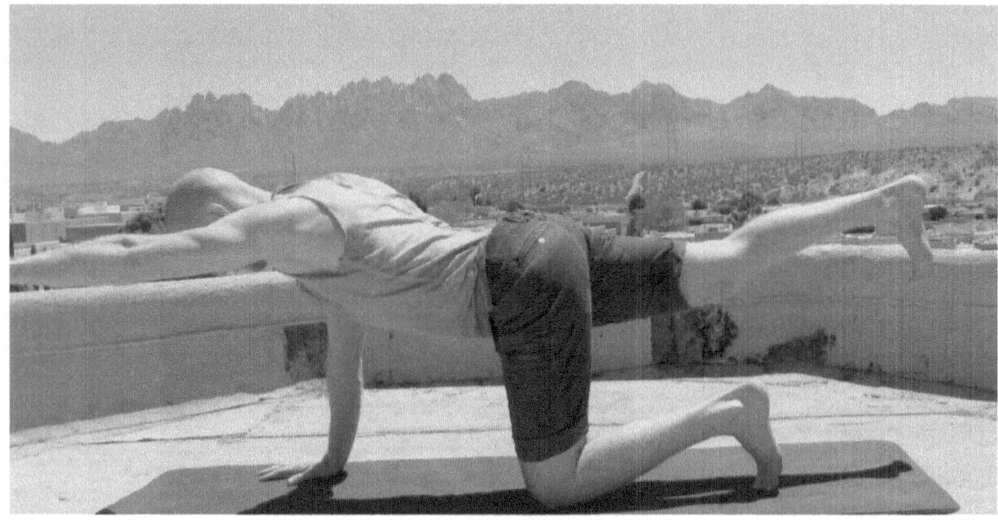

Stretch your right heel back like you're trying to press it into a wall. (The powerful valkyrie in the cover photo we chose is pointing her toes and lifting her head up, but actually the best form is to keep your head neutral, looking down at the floor, and flexing your toes!) Take care that your right hip doesn't start to lift upward, twisting your low back. If the hip does rise, bring it back down level with the left hip, but make sure you're still lifting the leg, really squeezing your right glutes. Keep the left arm raised, but keep the shoulder stable and locked into place by drawing your shoulder blade downward.

3. Hold your reps for no more than 7-8 seconds. Holding the posture for too long results in lack of available oxygen in your torso muscles. The result? Instability, and increased risk of aggravating your pain.

Switch sides with each rep.

CHAPTER FIFTEEN

Plank Variations

The classic plank is a powerful tool for strengthening your core muscles, whilst side planks are great for integrating your quadratus lumborum muscles and forcing them to work with your core to help stabilize your spine.

1. Start on all fours like you did in the previous posture, then come down to your elbows and straighten your legs. Grab hold of your elbows, and make sure your feet are about shoulder-width apart. Ease your heels back towards the rear of your yoga mat, whilst *strongly* engaging your abdominal brace. Squeeze your glutes, and make sure to draw your shoulders down away from your ears.

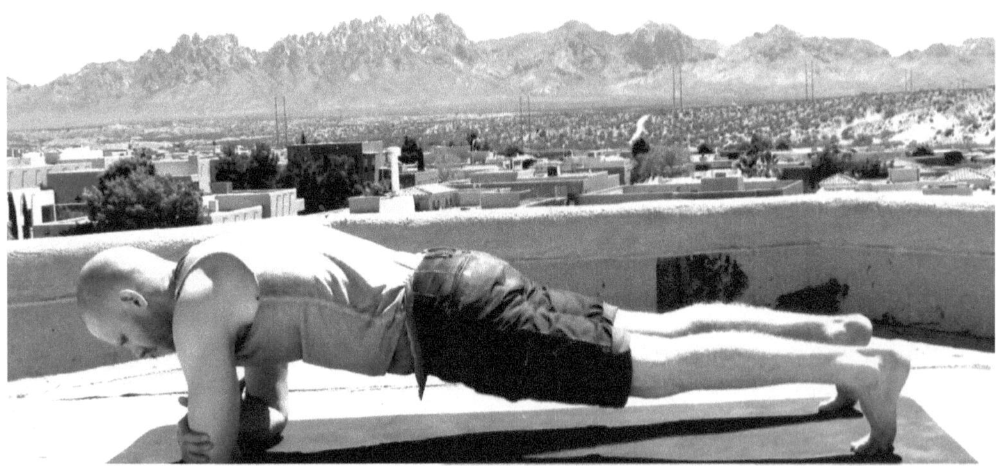

2. Hold this classic plank position for 8 seconds. It's vitally important not to get too aggressive with the duration.

Once you've mastered the classic plank and you're sure it's not provoking your back pain, you can transition from the classic plank into the Side Plank position…

3. The transition is probably the most tricky part, because the tendency is to initiate the roll into Side Plank your side from the *hips*, which essentially causes a miniature spine twist to occur in the lower back. Obviously, we're trying to avoid that, so instead of initiating the movement from the hips, I want you to initiate from the *shoulder*.

In order to roll onto your right side, make sure that in the classic Plank position you're still strongly pulling both shoulders down away from your ears, to keep your *latissimus dorsi* muscles engaged. Then, roll your left shoulder up on top of the right shoulder. If you have some shoulder issues, you can grab hold of that right shoulder with your left hand to help support the joint as your roll up. Notice that as you roll onto your right shoulder your left foot stays in front of the right foot.

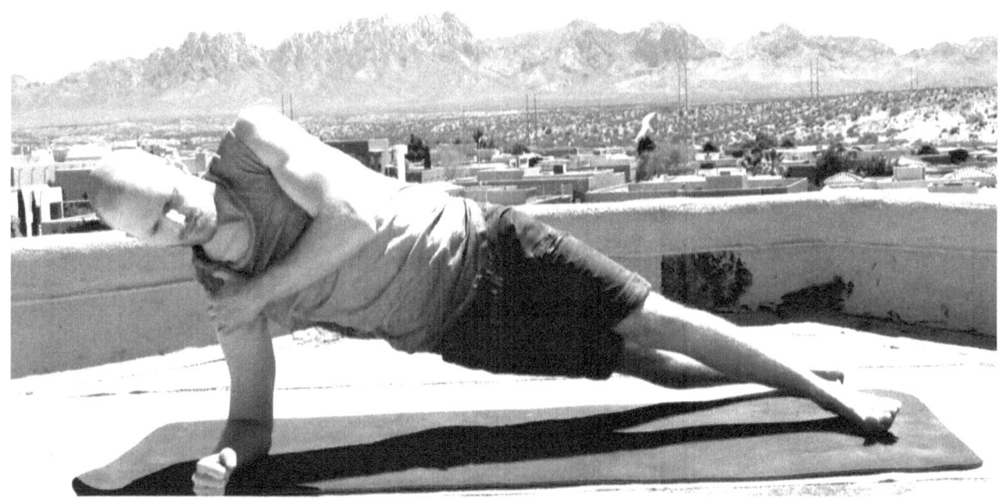

4. Keep pulling that right elbow towards your right hipbone to maintain a strong *lat* contraction. Keep the strongest abdominal brace you can manage, 100% effort, while still maintaining a calm, slow breath in and out through your nose, for 8 seconds.

5. To slightly increase the loading, you may place your left hand on your left hip.

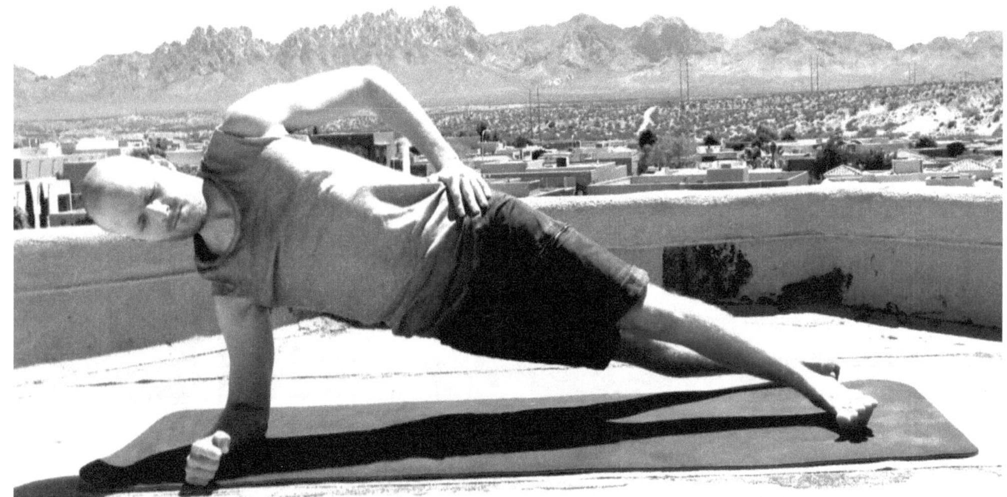

6. Now transition back to the classic Plank position, making sure to initiate the movement from the shoulder, not the hips.

Hold for an eight count, then repeat Side Plank on the other side by shoulder-initiating a roll onto your left elbow.

NOTE(S): If you find that Side Plank is too difficult, or seems to provoke back or shoulder pain, try this variation, with your knees stacked on top of each other:

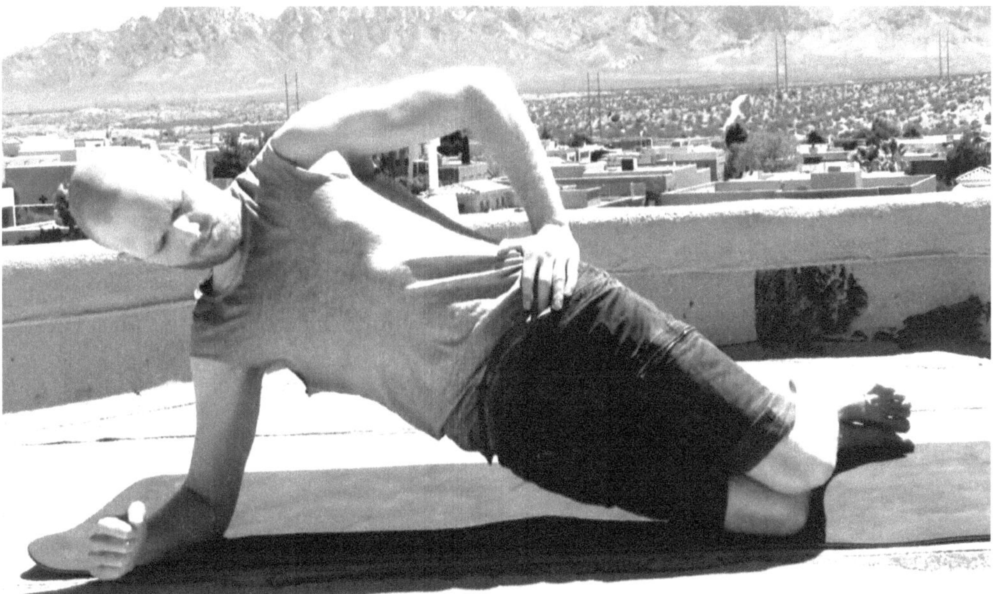

Remember, each Plank should only be held for 8 seconds before either a short rest, or transitioning to Side Plank.

In *Ultimate Back Fitness and Performance* (p.227) Dr. McGill writes that postures like this "should be held no longer than seven or eight seconds. The duration is based on recent evidence form near infrared spectroscopy indicating rapid loss of available oxygen in torso muscles contracting at these levels. Short relaxation of the muscle restores oxygen. The endurance objectives are achieved by building up repetitions of the exertions rather than increasing the duration of each hold."

It's up to you how many reps you want to do. Go nuts, as long as you're not getting aggressive with your hold times!

CHAPTER SIXTEEN

McGill Curl-Ups

This exercise, developed by Dr. McGill, is an excellent spine-sparing alternative to traditional crunches and abdominal exercises, which tend to promote pain-provoking spinal flexion and perpetuate harmful movement patterns.

1. Lie on your back with one leg bent and one leg straight, then layer your palms—one on top of the other—beneath your natural lumbar curve. This is important, as your hands will provide feedback and let you know if your lumbar spine is collapsing even the slightest bit during the exercise.

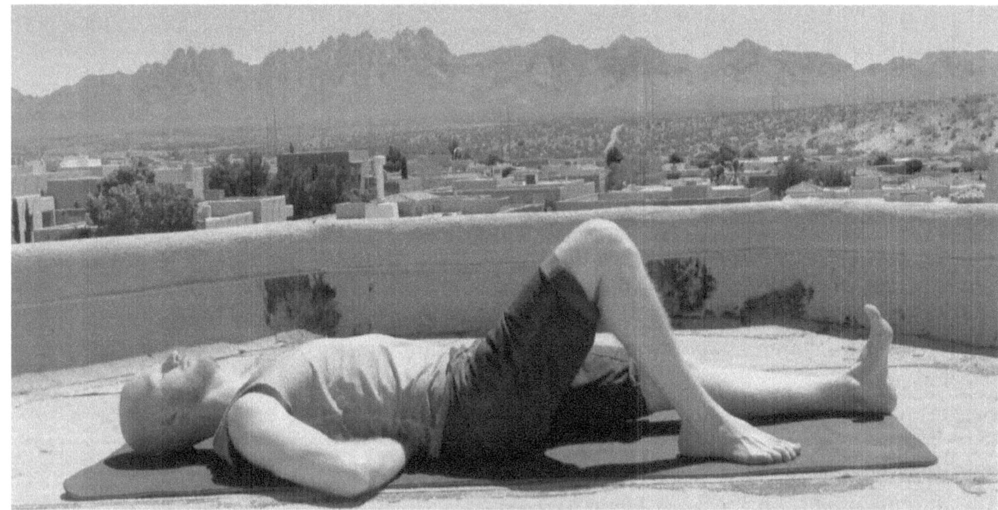

2. Now lift your elbows up off the floor, this will prevent you from "cheating" by using the elbows as a lever with which to initiate the curl up, which can tend to happen for beginners, especially if your core is weak and heretofore under-trained. But don't worry, this process will help you get those spine-protecting washboard abs in no time.

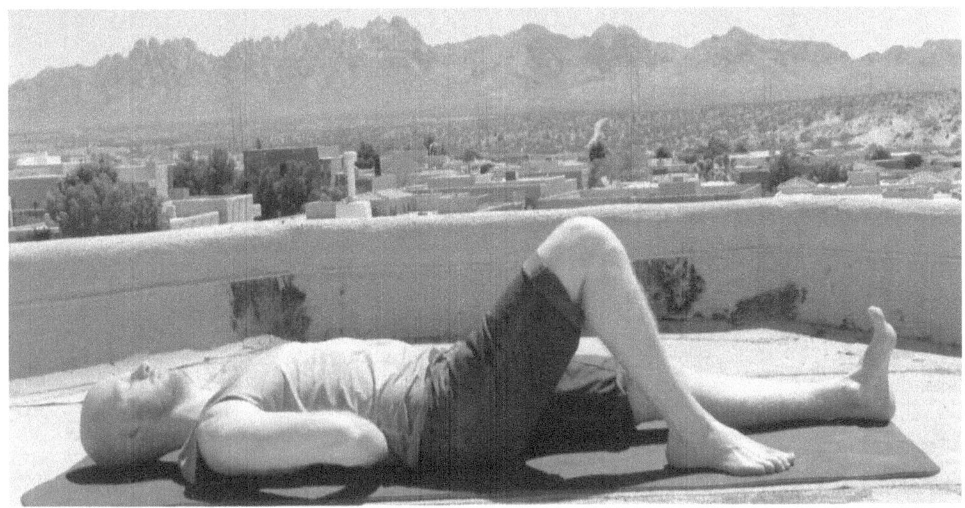

3. Here's where it gets tricky. The next step is to pretend you've got a scale directly beneath your head and shoulders. "Crunch up" by engaging your abs 100%, the idea being to lift your head and shoulders until the scale weighs zero. You're **not** actually going to lift your shoulders off the floor, and your head is *barely* going to lift up, only far enough to slide a piece of paper underneath. As you crunch up, if you feel your spine start to press down against your fingers, you're letting your low back collapse into spinal flexion and need to stop. Perform a 10 second hold *without* allowing your lumbar spine to move so much as a millimeter!

In the picture below, I'm doing it how beginners tend to want to do it. I'm lifting my head up too far, and I'm allowing my lumbar curve to collapse down against my fingers. Don't let this happen! While actively engaged in the posture, it should look *exactly* like step 2.

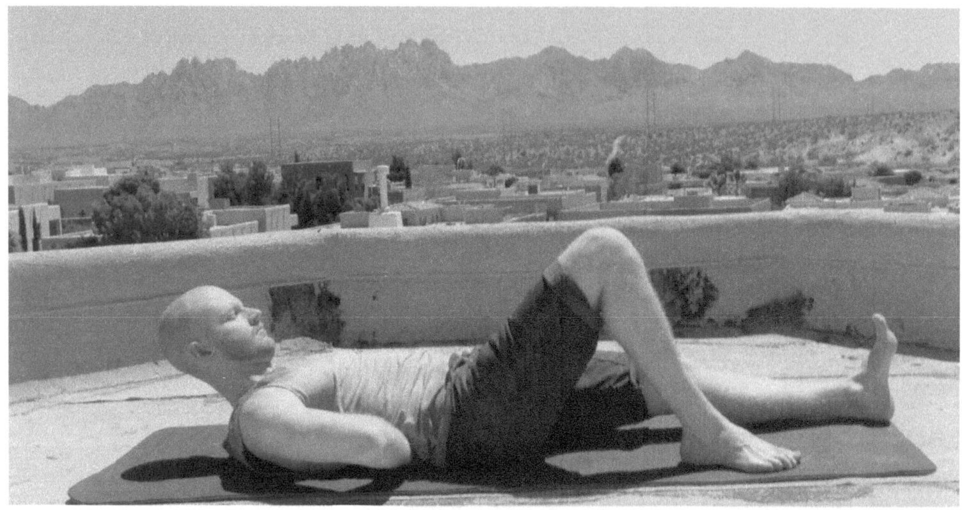

4. Switch legs and do the same thing on the other side. Hold for 8 seconds. Start with 4 total reps, build up from there. This is insanely fatiguing on the abs so don't overdo it. This is a great exercise for building endurance and strength.

NOTE: This is one of the few postures in which I *don't* advocate calm, slow breathing through the nose. A strong exhalation through the mouth seems to work best, at least for me. I begin each rep with a deep inhale through the nose, then slowly exhale through the mouth, like blowing through a straw, for the full 8 seconds of the posture hold.

McGill Curl-Ups + Neurological Pulsing

This variation of the Curl-Up, also developed by Dr. McGill, trains your spine to stay braced and neutral during sudden hip flexion. That makes this a great drill to perform if you would like to integrate running into your exercise program once your back starts feeling better.

1. Start in the basic Curl-Up position, but whichever leg is straight, bring the *opposite* arm up over your head.

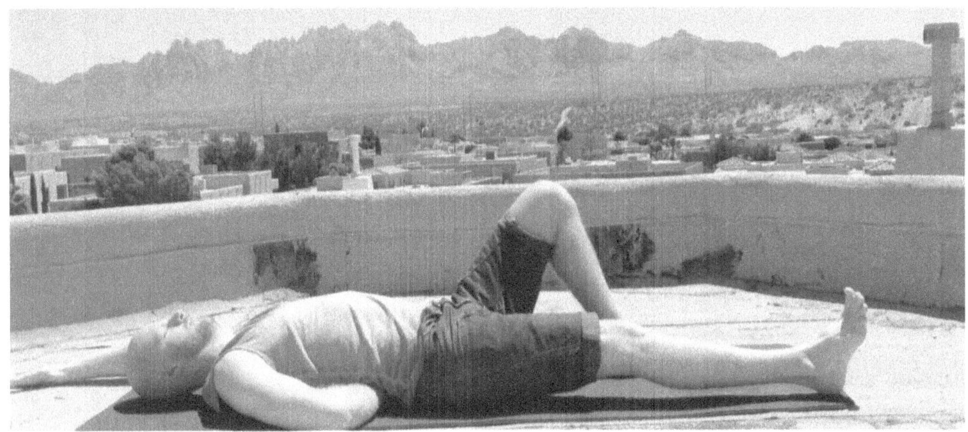

2. Now 'pulse up' with that arm and leg.

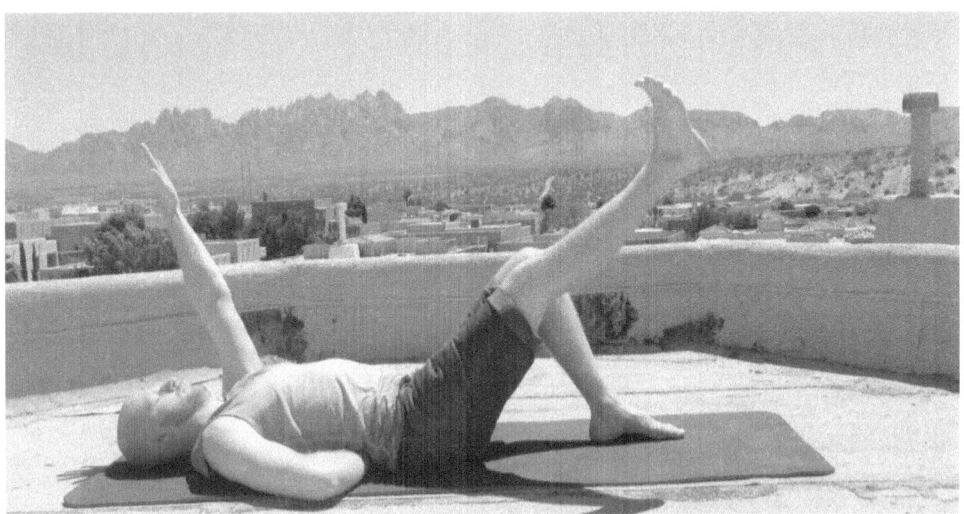

3. Pulse upward as quickly as possible, bringing the arm to about shoulder level, and the leg up to roughly the level of your opposite knee. Then, quickly lower your arm and leg back down to the start position. Perform three quick pulses.

4. For your next set of three pulses, bring the arm and leg up about half the distance you did the first time.

5. For your final set of three, pulse up just barely off the floor.

6. Then switch sides and repeat the whole drill of 9 total pulses with the other arm and leg.

Just like in the Curl-Up, make sure your lower back doesn't collapse into flexion as you perform your pulses. We're still training Braced Neutral Spine position here, but we're also training controlled hip flexion and neurological quickness. Think: "Proximal Stiffness, Distal Quickness!" In other words, tight and protected core, fast and supple movement of the limbs.

CHAPTER SEVENTEEN

Bridge

Many of us who struggle with back pain are not helped by the fact that our gluteal muscles have become, essentially, *lazy.*

Too much sitting is problematic not just because of spinal flexion and compression, but the constant compression of the gluteal muscles can cause deactivation, at which point the muscles get very lackadaisical about doing their job properly. Combine that with chronically shortened hip flexors, and you get mechanical inhibition of end-range hip extension, which can make it difficult to open up your hips and leaves you with a multitude of issues: lazy glutes *and* hip pain to go along with your back pain, creating this feedback loop of chronic discomfort and dysfunction.

Bridge pose specifically targets weak glutes and tight hip flexors in a way that I have found to be generally well-tolerated by yoga practitioners struggling with low back pain. However, it can be easy to 'cheat.' There is often a tendency for the hamstrings to want to take over from the poor, sleepy glutes, to the point that hamstrings wind up doing *all* the work, the glutes never wanting to engage. I'll show you how to avoid that pitfall.

1. Start on your back with your feet flat, maintaining a gentle abdominal brace and the same neutral curve in the low back that we practiced maintaining in the McGill Curl-Ups previously.

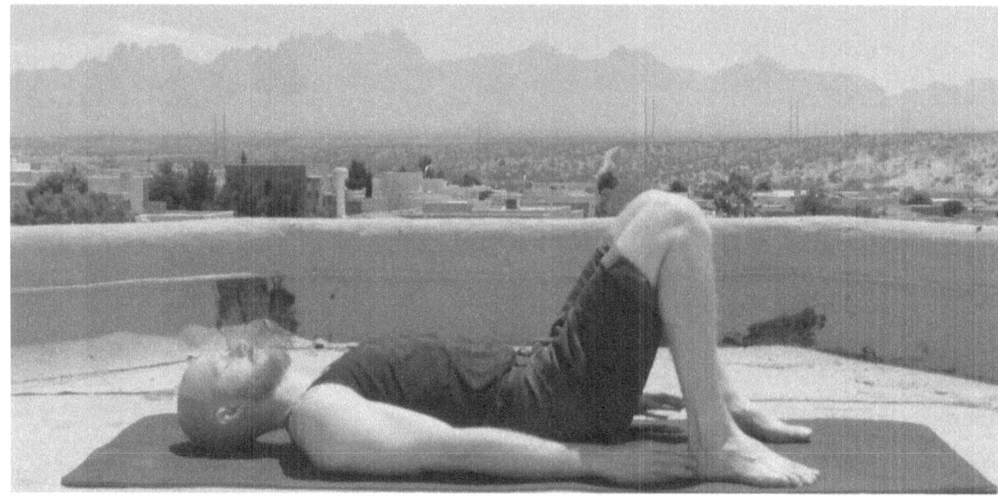

2. Maintain your Braced Neutral spine but squeeze your glutes as hard as you can, maximum contraction, and press down through your *heels* to lift your hips off the floor, getting your hips into as much extension as possible.

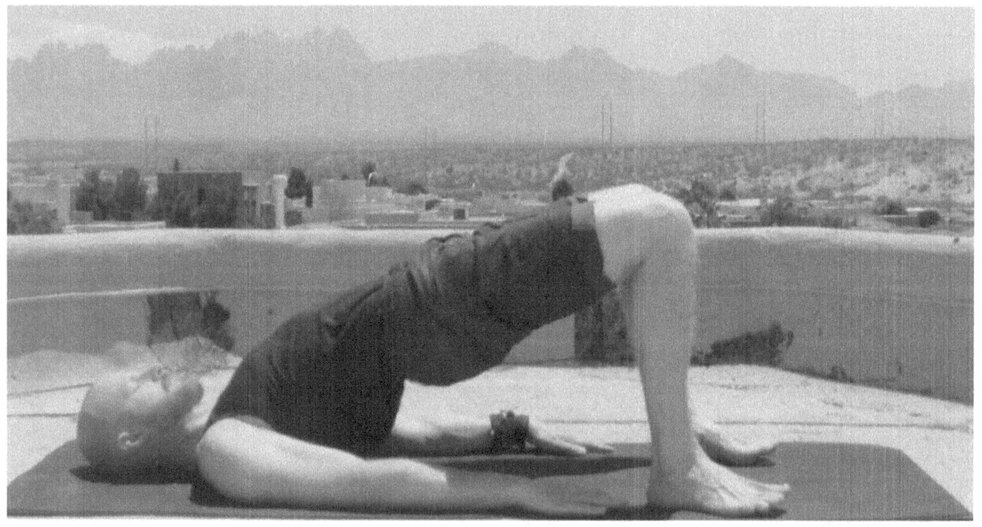

Hold for 8 seconds, then let your hips return to the floor for a quick rest before performing the next rep.

To avoid hamstring 'cheating', see if you can lift your toes and the balls of your feet off your yoga mat during the posture, so only the heels remain in contact with the floor. Perform 4 repetitions to begin with, slowly adding reps as you get stronger.

Remember to always focus on locking down your spinal joints. Don't let your spine break from Braced Neutral at any point.

NOTE: I don't want to over-coach the breathing here. I find that every student likes to breathe a little differently. Some students like to take a big inhale to start, then slowly exhaling for an 8 count, which may help pressurize your abdomen and maintain Braced Neutral. Other students like to exhale up and slowly inhale for an 8 count. Still others like to maintain a calm flow of 4 count inhales and 4 count exhales during this pose. Find what works best for you.

3. When you find your comfort zone with Bridge, you can graduate to the one-legged version. Press up through both heels, then once you've reached maximum hip extension, lift one leg straight up in the air, flexing your toes towards your face.

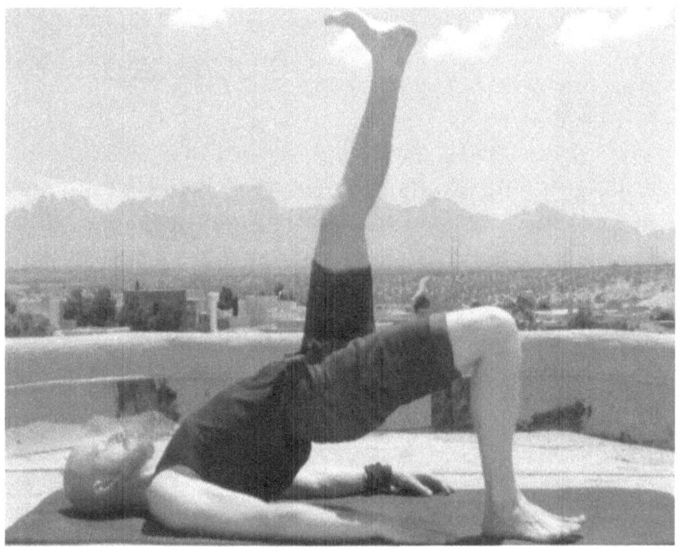

NOTE(S): This one-leg version may aggravate sciatica in some students, so please be mindful and avoid this variation if it provokes your pain.

Also, this is about as close as we ever come to getting a hamstring 'stretch' in this sequence, but please do not overdo it. If you feel too much of a stretch, back off. You'll notice in the preceding photo that while my toes are flexed, my knee is bending slightly. Locking out the knee will increase the hamstring stretch and is unnecessary.

Please remember that 'tight hamstrings' likely have nothing to do with your pain. That's a popular myth in the yoga community. In fact, 'tight' hammies will aid in your athletic performance! In *Ultimate Back Fitness and Performance* (p.12), Dr. McGill writes that "hamstrings contribute shearing stability to the knee such that lengthening them has been reported to be associated with elevated disruption of the anterior cruciate ligament. No wonder the bulk of the literature has shown no link between hamstring tightness and back pain, either current pain or predicting future pain."

CHAPTER EIGHTEEN

Passive Thoracic Extension

This simple posture is designed to help correct rounding in the upper back, called 'kyphosis,' which is common as people age, but which has become quite common among young people as well, thanks to so much time slouched over computers and phones. This directly effects the lower back by over-activating the spinal muscles, so it's never wise to ignore the upper back when low back pain is present.

As a bonus, this posture also helps your shoulders function more efficiently.

I've tried to avoid using props as much as possible, but for this posture you will need a stool, chair, or some other elevated platform on which to rest your elbows.

1. Start on your knees, placing your elbows on the edge of the platform, then bringing your palms together in prayer position. You can then bring your palms back towards your shoulder blades as far as they can go. There's no need to brace your spine here, just relax into the stretch as much as possible, letting your chest sink towards the floor. Hold here for at least one minute.

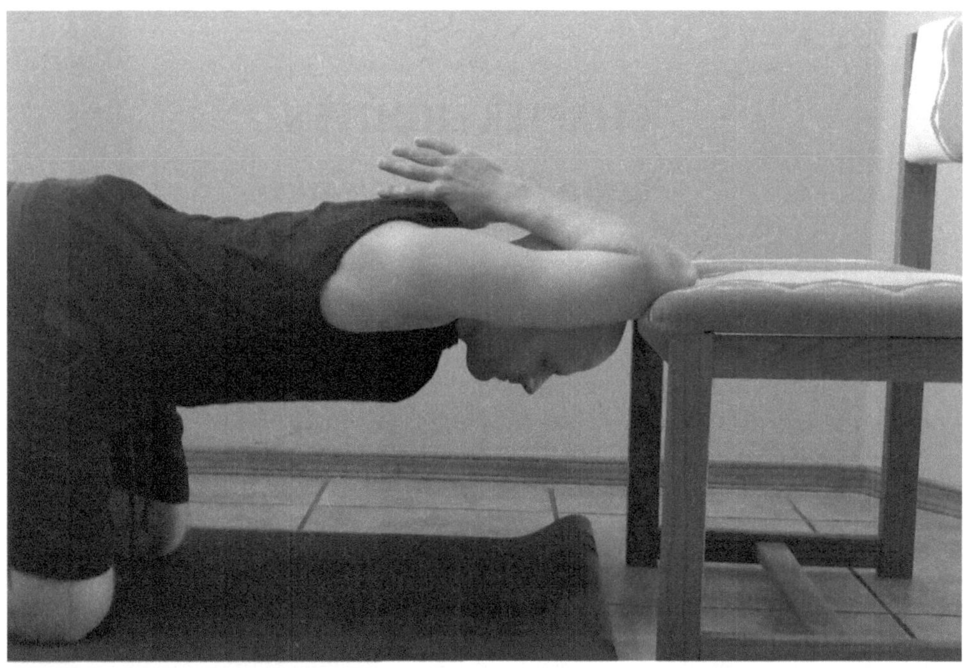

NOTE: To intensify the stretch, you can take a deep inhale and press your elbows down against the platform with moderate effort, hold for about 5 seconds, then exhale and relax. You may find that you sink even more deeply into thoracic extension by using this contract-relax technique.

CHAPTER NINETEEN

Turkish Get-Ups

The Turkish Get-Up is perhaps the most complex movement pattern in this entire series.

There are *many* different versions of this exercise, so those of you who are familiar with this exercise may find that I coach the Get-Up rather differently than you're accustomed to.

It will become clear rather quickly that the Get Up is best left alone until your lower back pain has been substantially diminished, and for the casual practitioner I would say this section is entirely optional. However, for those of you itching to rehabilitate your back so that you can return to the gym or resume playing a sport, I think this exercise is key. Dr. McGill has said of the Get Up, "For many athletes, learning to lock the ribcage on the pelvis is essential for injury prevention and performance…A terrific exercise for transitioning into performance is the Turkish Get up, where the spine posture is controlled and the overhead weight is steered as the body learns more movement strategies that maintain torso stiffness while driving with other extremities." (http://www.robotfightfitness.com/2013/06/10/turkish-get-up/)

I will show you how to do each step of the Get-Up *without* a kettlebell. When learning the movement, always start without a kettlebell and only progress to the weighted version after you have mastered every stage, pain-free.

NOTE: A good intermediate step between weighted and un-weighted, which encourages stability, is to perform the entire Turkish Get-Up with a shoe balanced on your closed fist, like so…

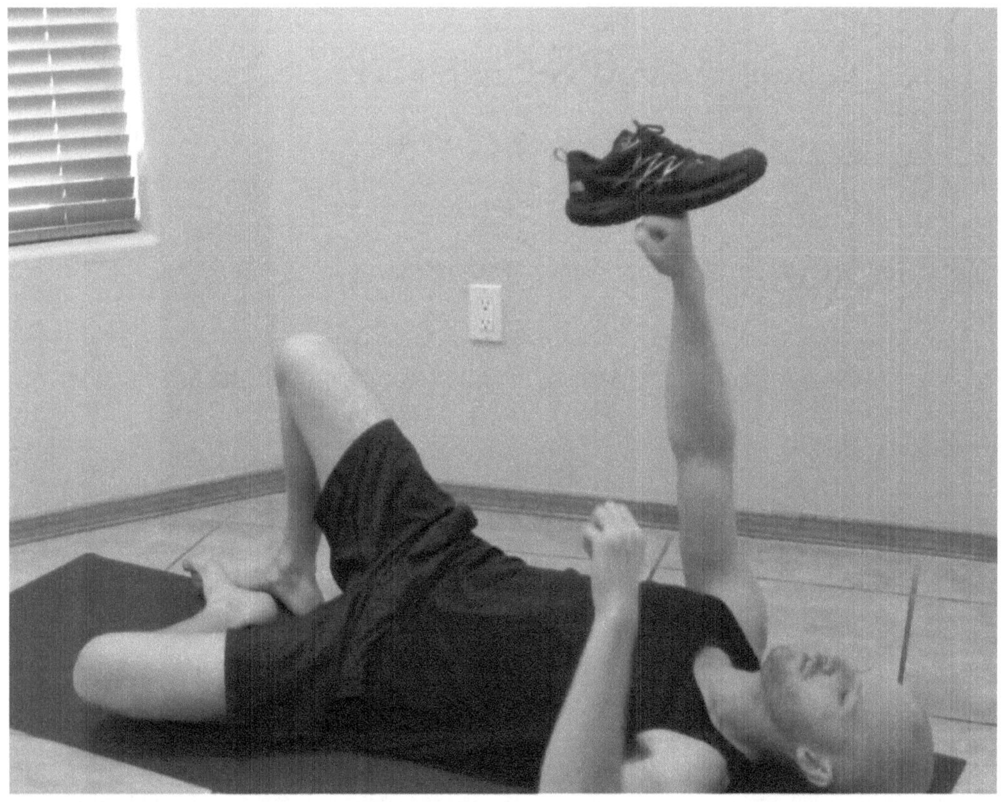

Once you've mastered this, and can get all the way through without the shoe falling off, you're probably ready to load the movement with a very modest weight. But first we'll learn the unweighted version:

1. Start by lying on your back with a braced neutral spine, your legs in the 'clamshell' position, and your arms positioned like so:

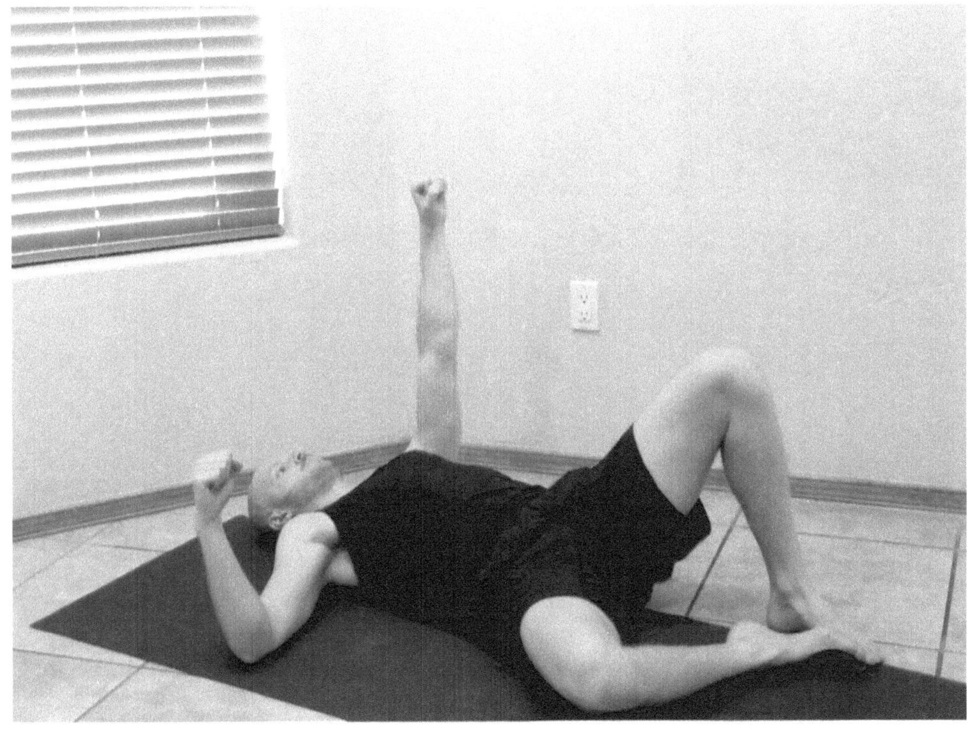

Start with your left arm straight up in the air. That's the arm that's going to be holding the 'imaginary' kettlebell, so that's the knee that you want pointing straight up.

2. Press your right elbow down into the floor (make sure to do this on a soft surface like a thick rubber yoga mat). I also want you to think about pulling that elbow slightly down towards your right hipbone. The elbow shouldn't actually travel down much lower than shoulder level, I just want you to feel the sensation of your right shoulder engaging here before you move on. This subtle engagement will help you keep your spine neutral as you move to the next step.

3. **Maintaining Braced Neutral spine position**, press down through your left heel, squeeze your left glutes and launch your left hip over top of your right hip, coming up on your right elbow.

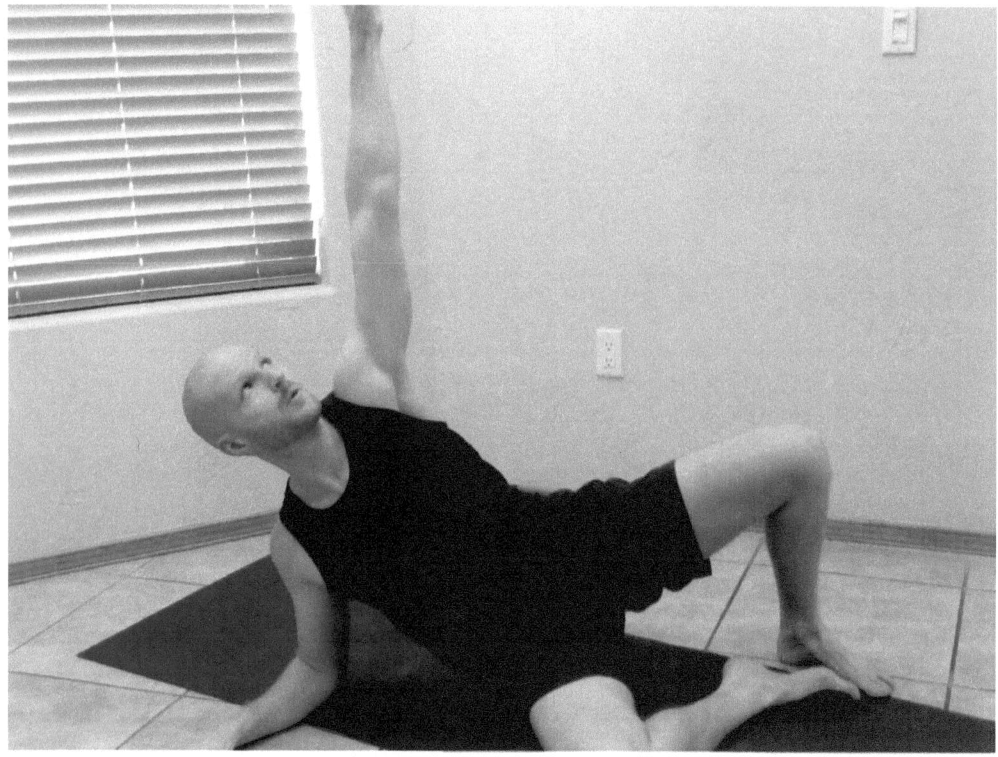

This is easily the most 'iffy' step, because the natural tendency is to want to engage the abs and 'crunch up' into this position. I don't want you to do that! Use your left glutes to propel you into this potion, without letting your low back collapse into flexion, not even a little bit. It's *not* a crunch or a sit-up!

4. Next you're going to straighten that right arm. It's good to get into the habit of staring up at your left hand because when you actually start holding a weight it's always a good idea to keep your eye on it!

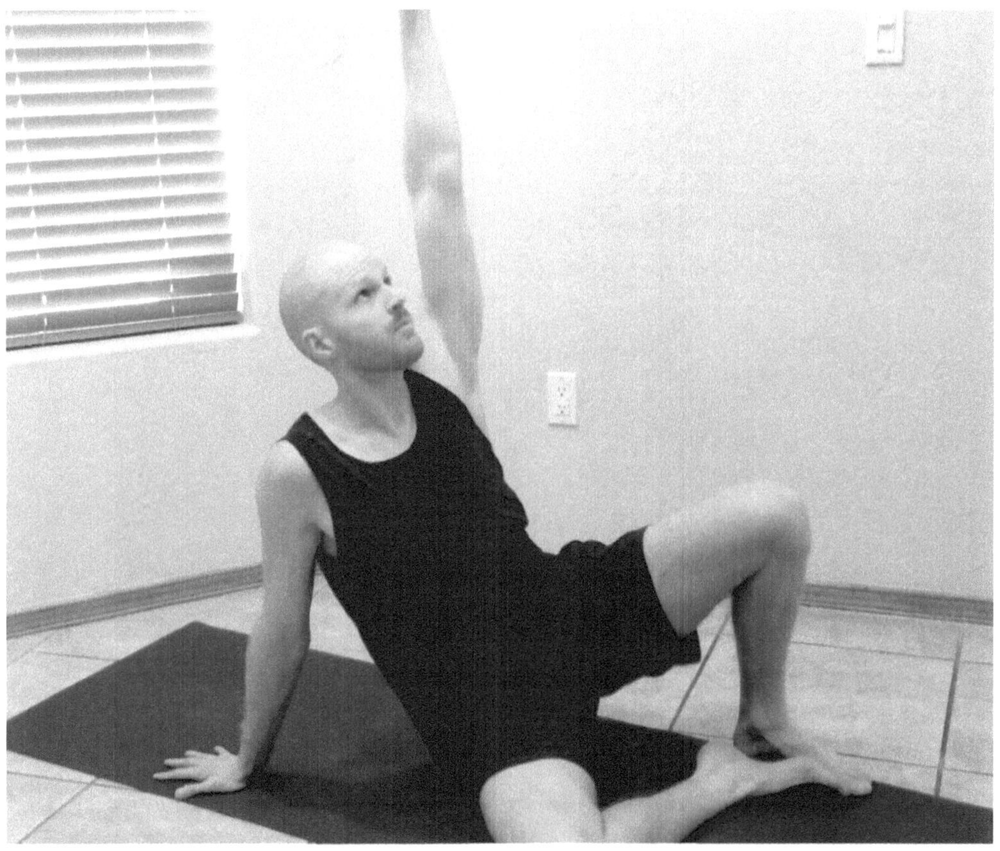

5. Now keep your abdomen braced and your chest lifted as you sweep that right knee back into a good position to transition up into your good Lunge pose. If your right knee comes tor rest directly behind your left heel, you won't be able to move into a good, balanced Lunge…

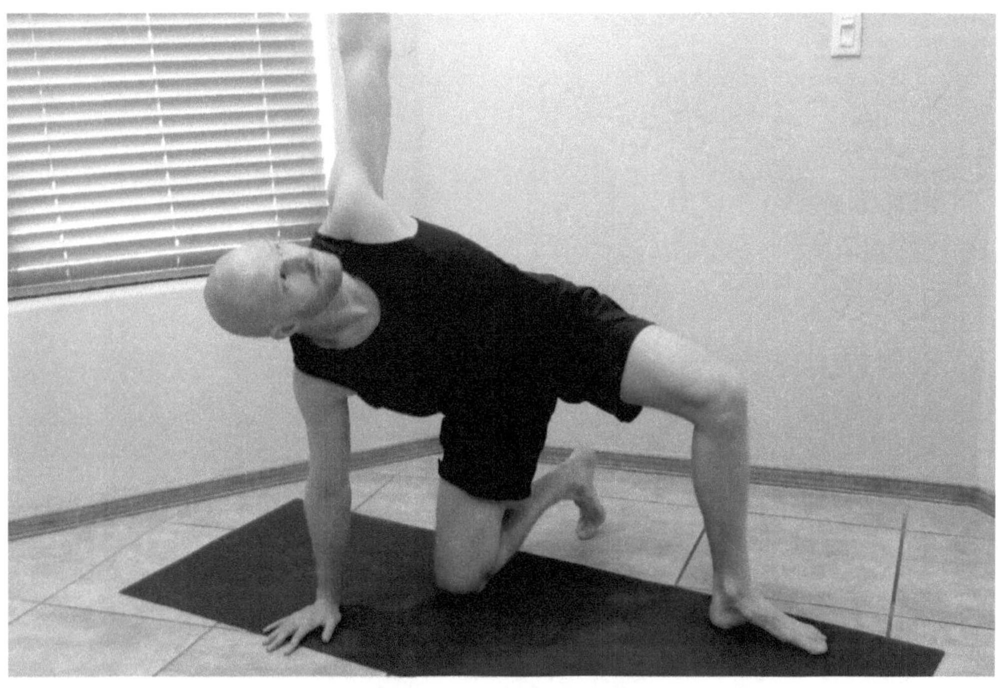

6. Now I want you to very slightly nudge your hips back towards your right heel, reconnect with your abdominal brace, then lift your torso up whilst "windshield-wipering" your back leg. This should bring you into a good, balanced Lunge...

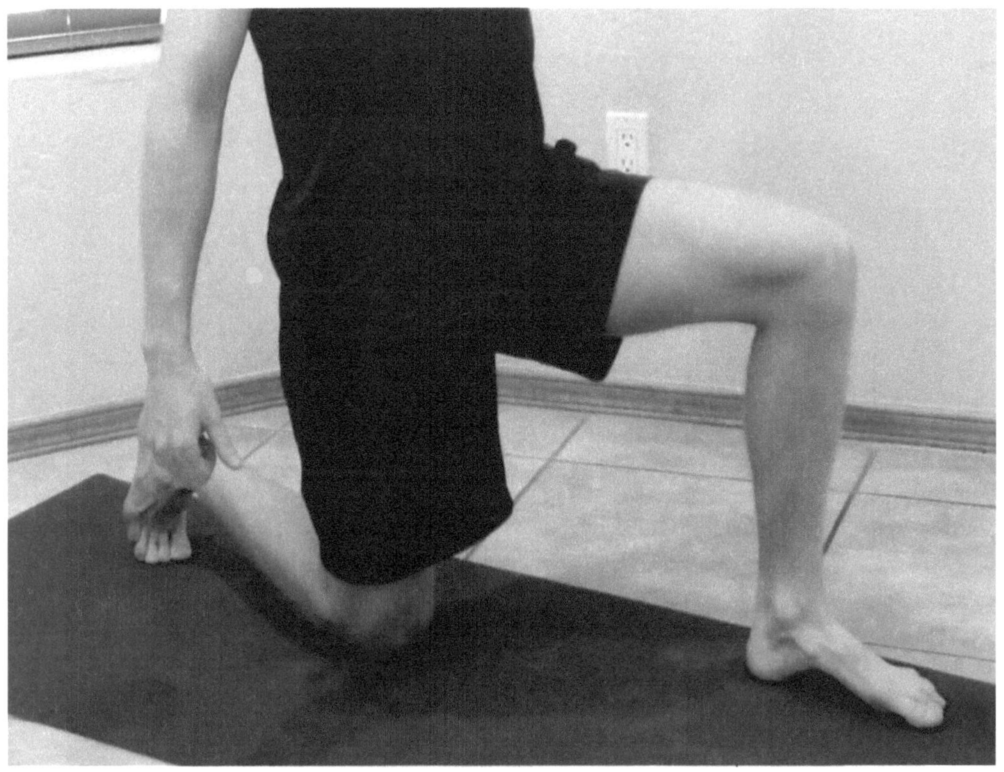

7. Now all you have to do is stand up, and pause for a calm breath at the top.

8. But you're only halfway done! From here, perform a reverse lunge, and simply reverse the steps to come back down to the start position:

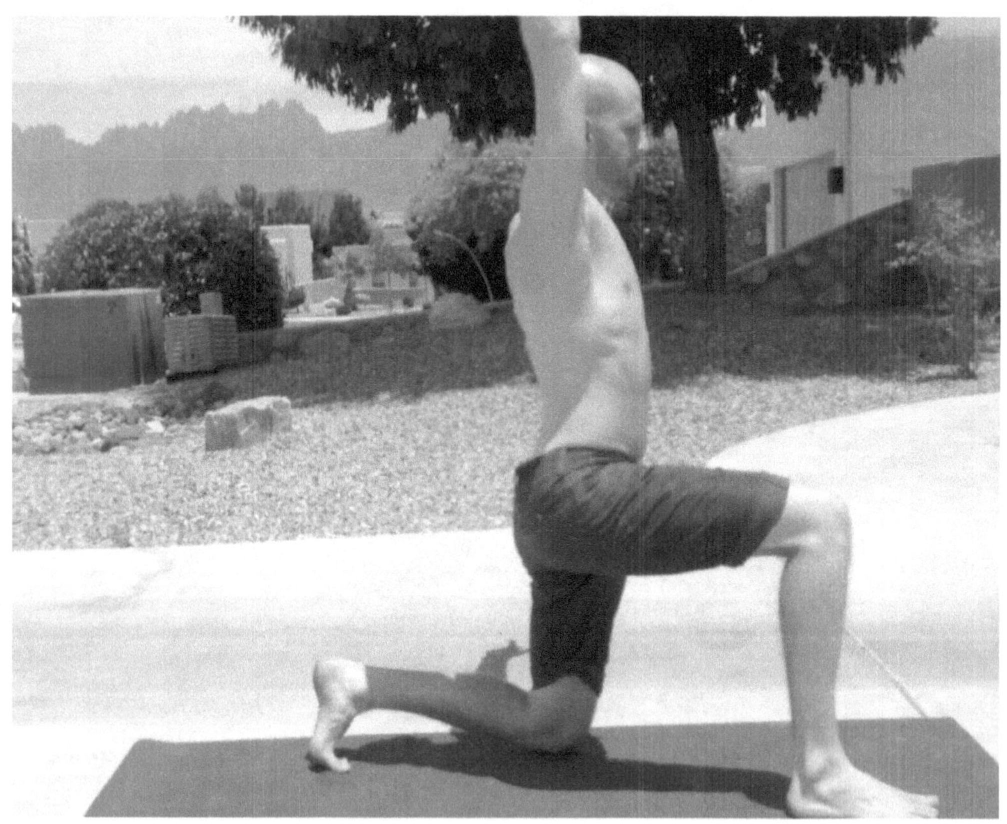

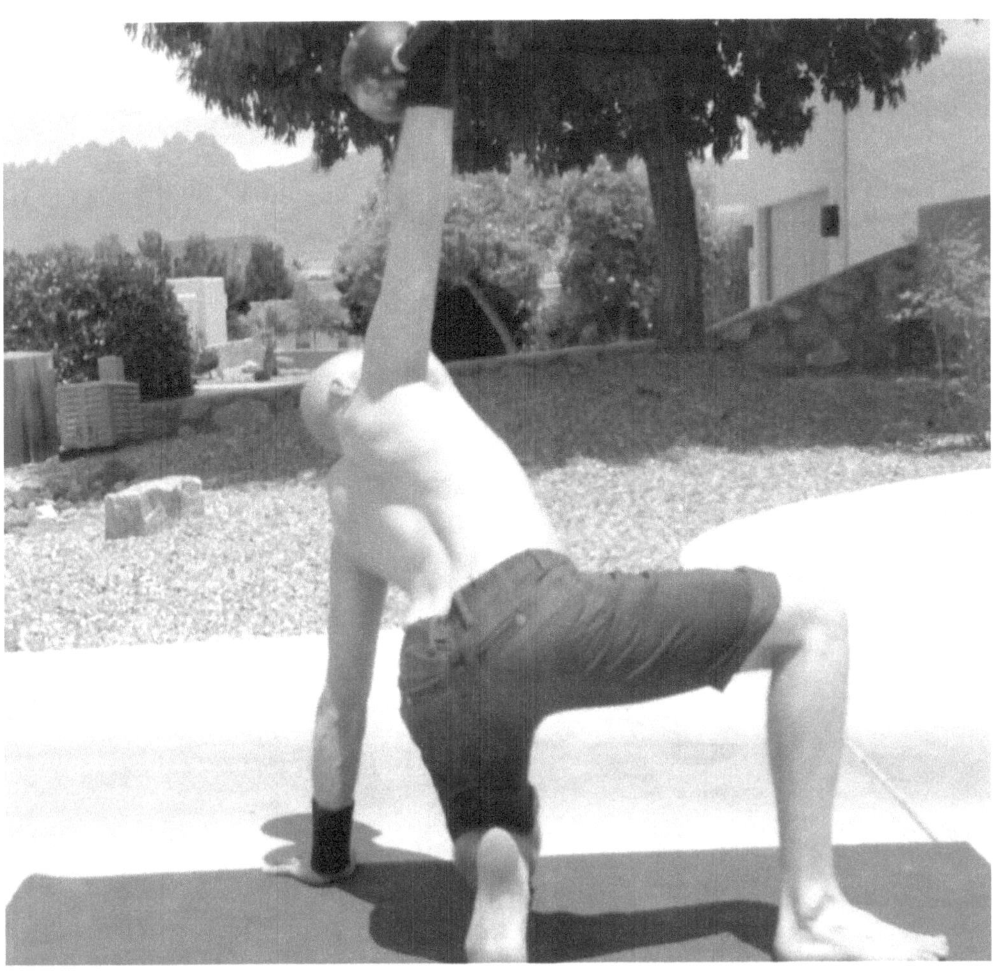

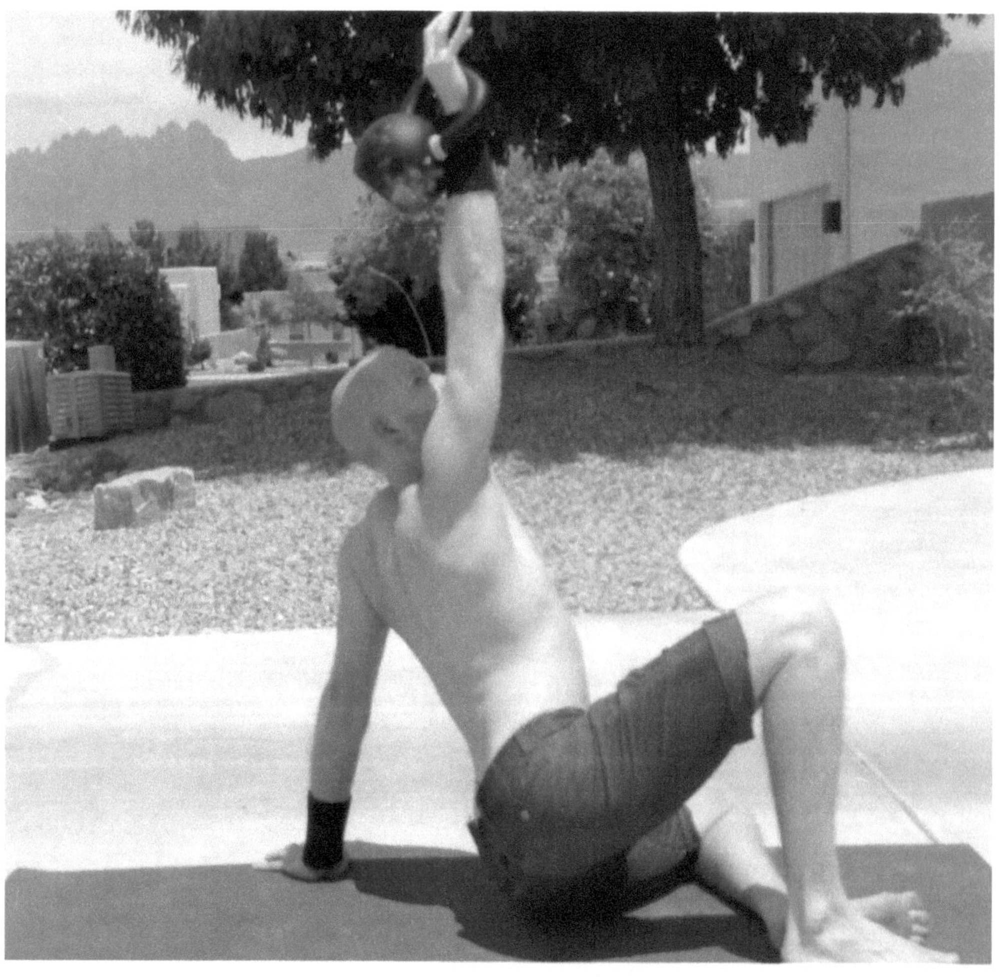

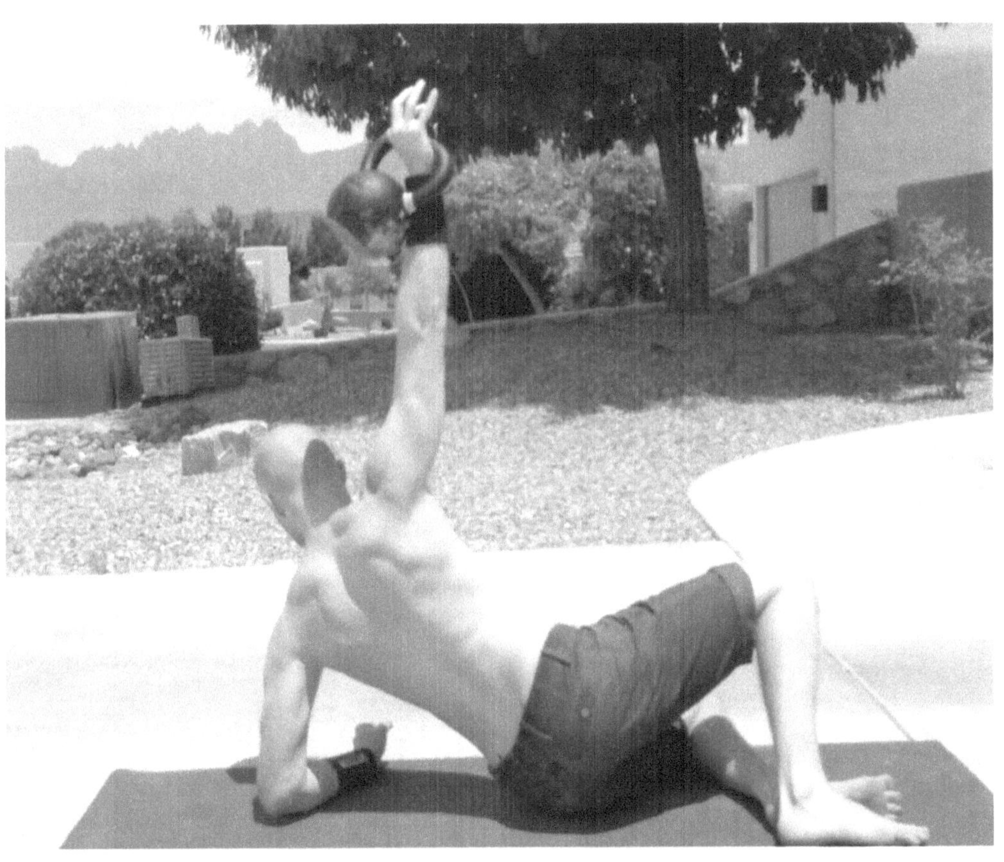

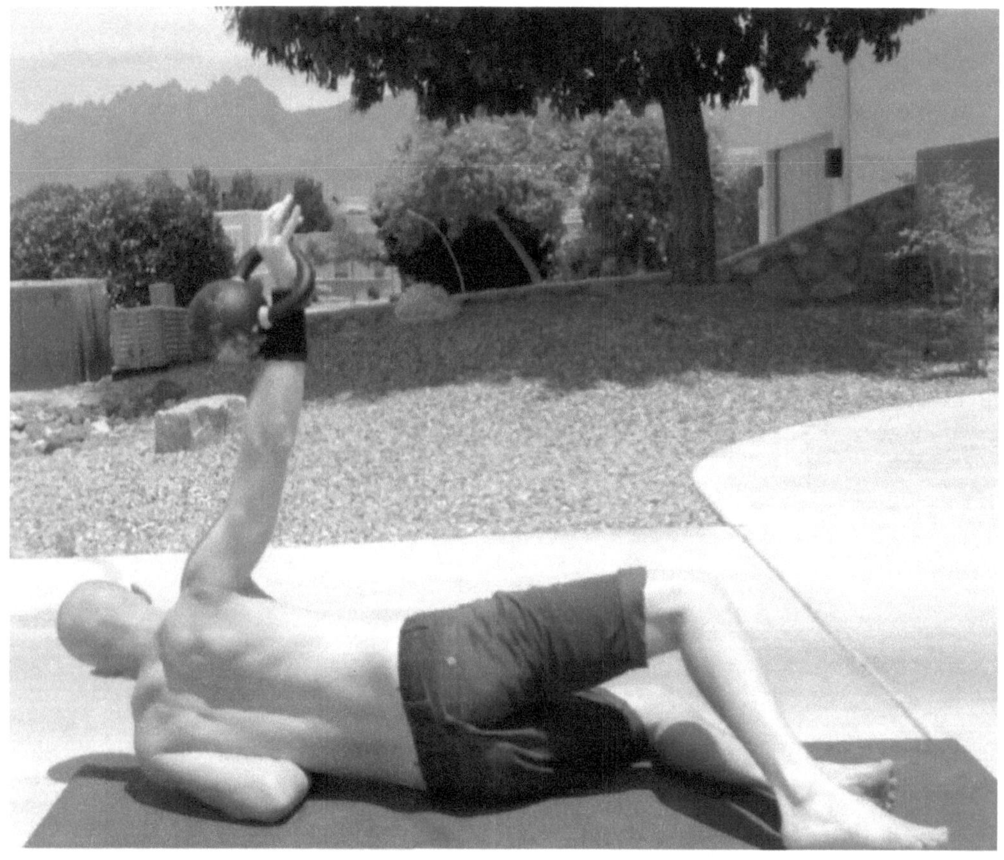

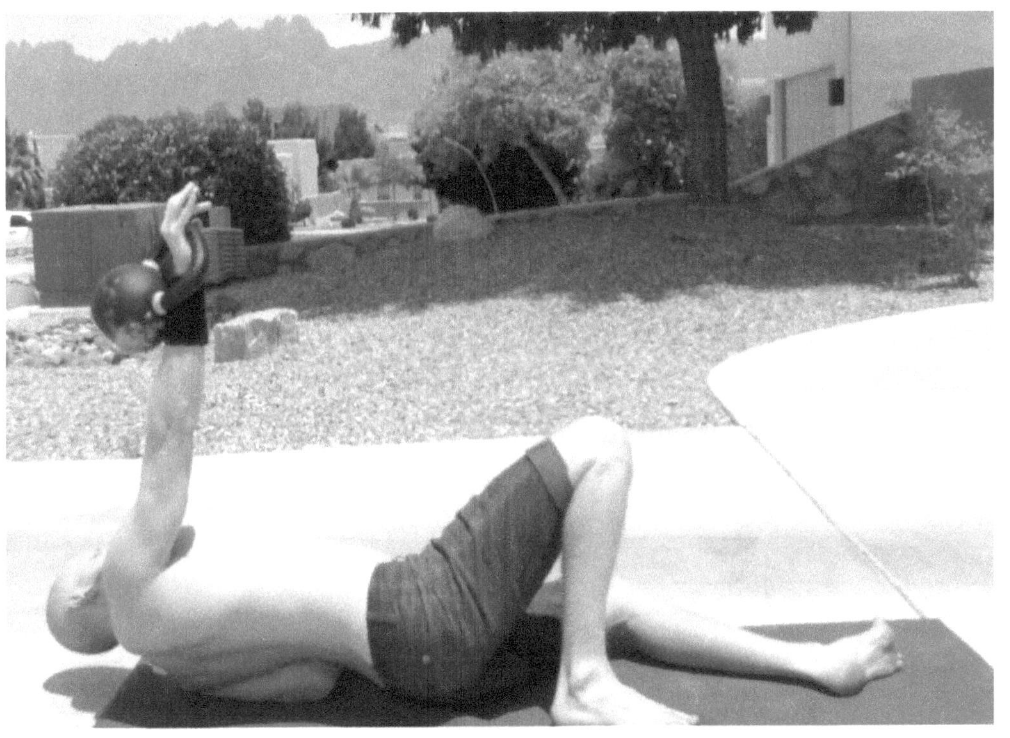

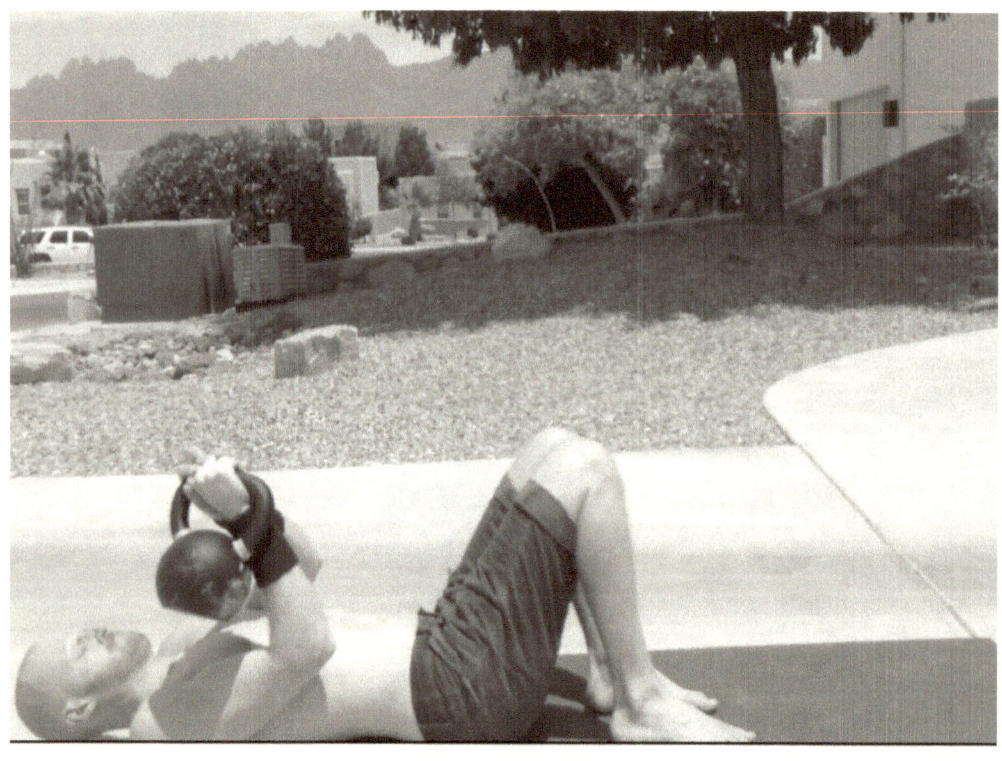

CHAPTER TWENTY

Kettlebell Carries

I've tried to keep this course firmly planted on the yoga mat, but the kettlebell carry is the exception. Even though practicing these will take you off the mat, I felt I would be remiss to exclude them from this course, because they're so great for building strength and endurance in your spine. Also, carries can offer a good alternative to Planks for those of you who find that our Plank variations are initially provocative to your pain. Besides which, Dr. McGill has said, "I consider that every general program to enhance athleticism needs a carry task." (https://www.backfitpro.com/documents/bottomupart.pdf)

Kettlebell carries particularly activate the quadratus lumborum muscles in your lower back, which are the muscles that go haywire in acute flare-ups of back pain that leave you unable to stand up straight, or walk without feeling like someone is stabbing you in the lower back. Those of you who have been reduced by your back pain to crawling to the bathroom on your hands and knees will know what it's like to have a dysfunctional quadratus lumborum.

Obviously, start with short carries, about 20-30 paces. I'm rather fond of finishing my yoga practice by walking around the block carrying my kettlebells, but it took me a long time to build up to that.

The most basic carries are the Single Arm and the Farmer's Carry. For the Single Arm Carry, simply pick up a kettlebell in one hand and carry it like you'd carry a bag of groceries. This will give you the benefits of asymmetrical loading, as the muscles on the contralateral side work overtime to stabilize you. Carry for a set number of paces, then switch arms and repeat.

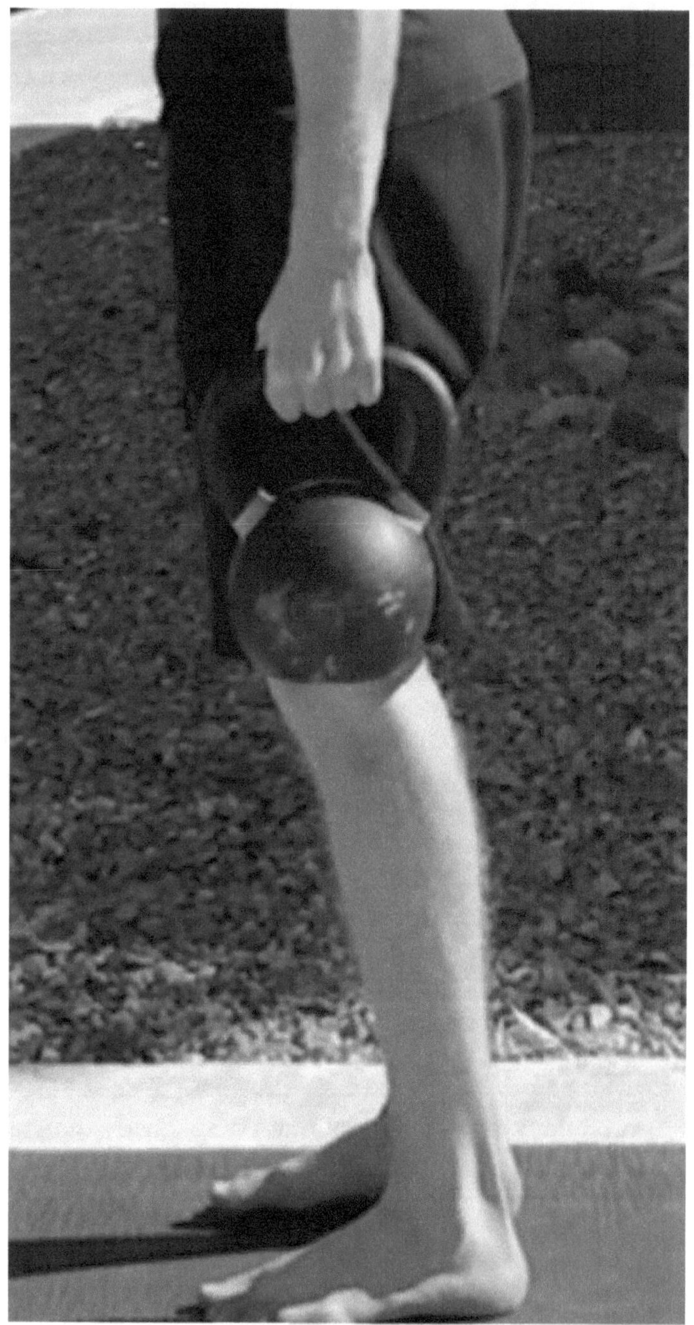

For the Farmer's Carry, walk with a kettlebell in each hand. You're losing the asymmetrical loading benefit, but you're basically doubling the compressive load so there are benefits and drawbacks to each. You may find Farmer's carries provocative to your pain, but be fine with Single Arm carries, or vice versa.

You can also do a Rack Carry:

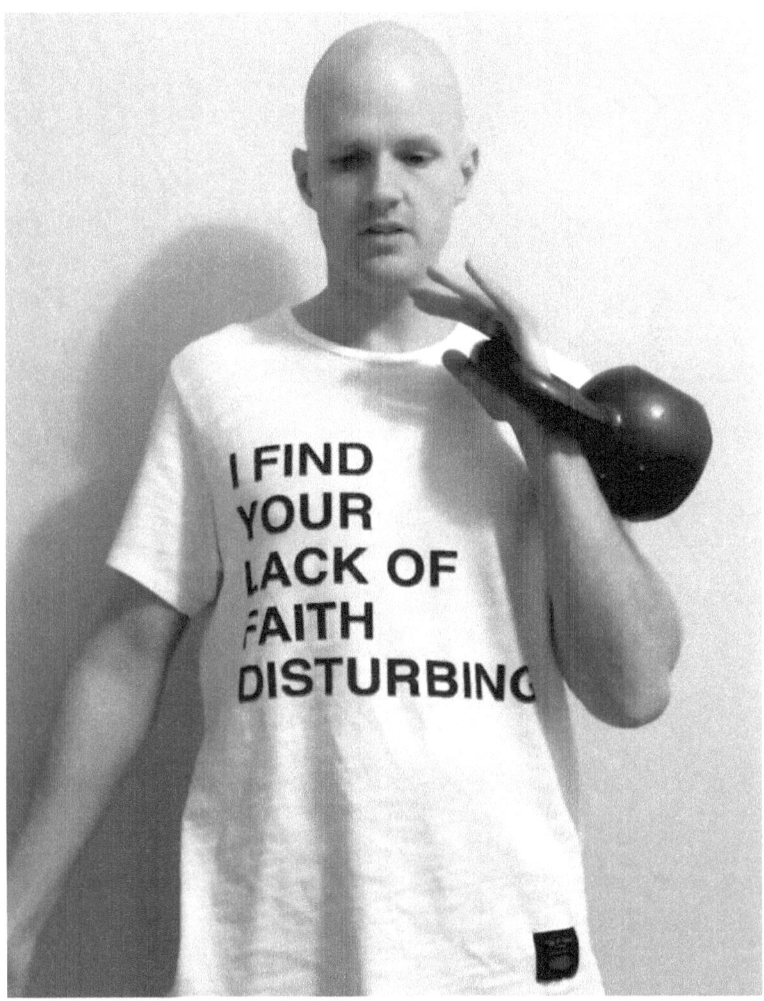

Another variation is the overhead carry, in which you first bring the kettlebell into the rack position, then press the kettlebell overhead:

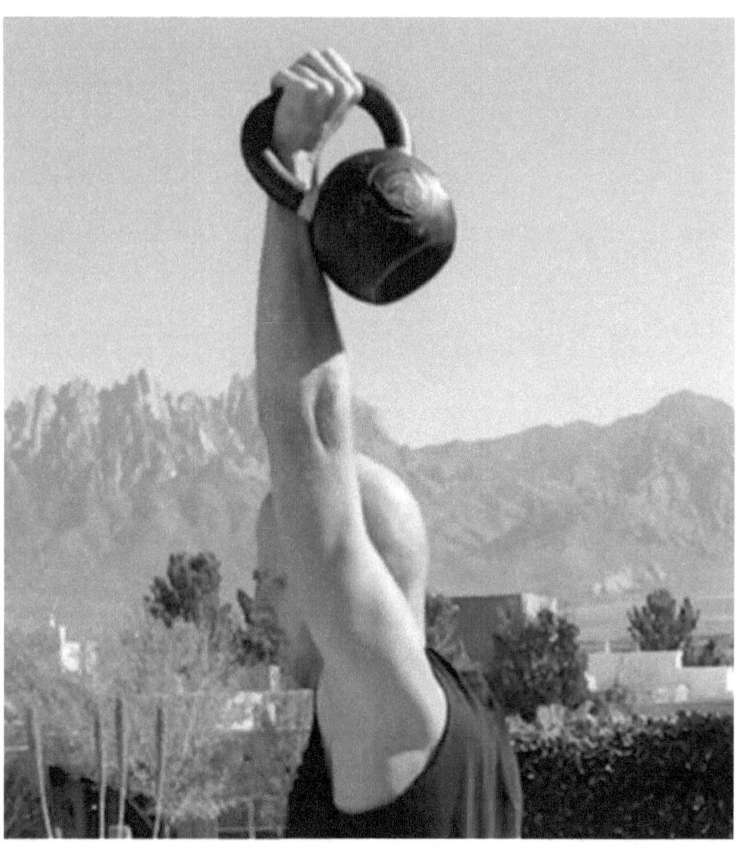

If you're going to do overhead carries, remember to keep your shoulder pulled down. If you press the bell over your head and find that suddenly you're wearing your shoulder like an earring, that's not a particularly stable position, so slide that shoulder down your back and lock it into place before you start walking your paces.

Perhaps the most effective carry for building stability and endurance is the single arm Bottom's Up Carry:

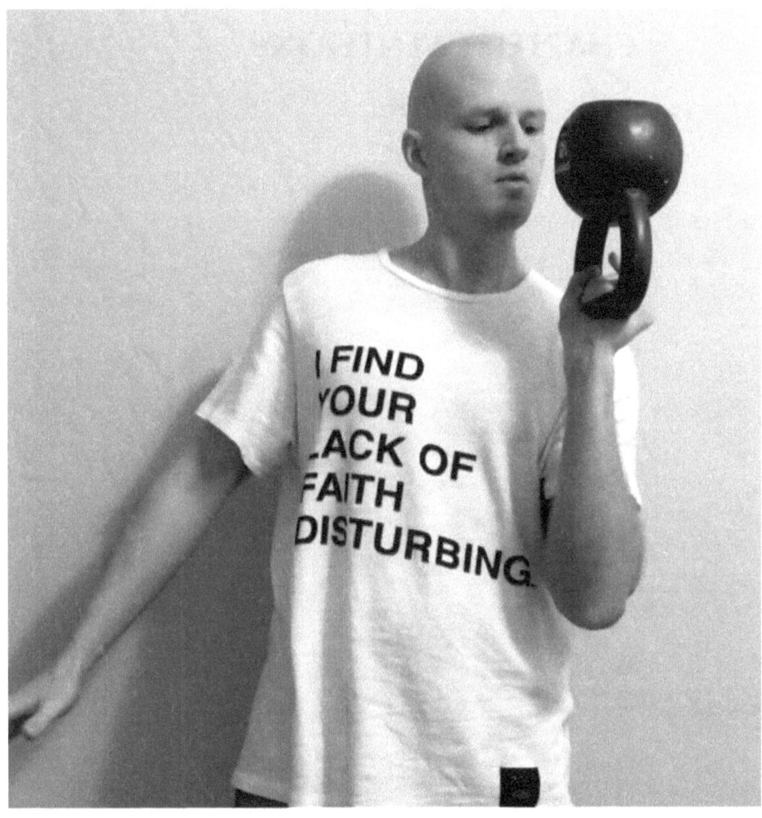

It can be helpful to chalk up your hands before you try this one! Wrist guards can also be helpful, because obviously if things go awry that kettlebell can fall out of position and whack you square on the wrist.

Notice how, in the preceding image, I've got my pinky finger elevated, like a proper lady drinking tea. That helps me keep the carry 'honest,' because a raised pinky makes it hard to maintain a death grip on the kettlebell, as a way of compensating for lack of stability.

CHAPTER TWENTY-ONE

Fixed Firm

The final posture in this sequence is a version of Fixed Firm pose. If you can begin by sitting on your heels for a few rounds of breathing, knees together, seiza-style, please do so.

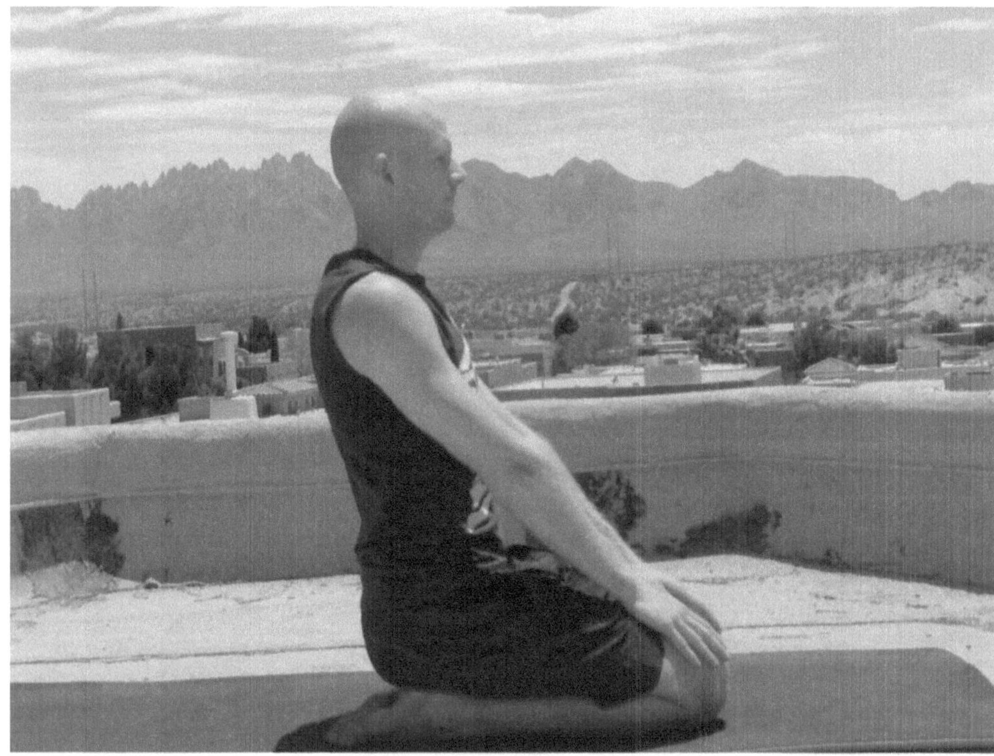

However, many students find this position impossible to achieve due to discomfort in the knees. If that's the case for you, separate your knees and heels then simply ease your hips back towards your heels as far as they can comfortably go without provoking knee pain, remembering to maintain a braced neutral spine position:

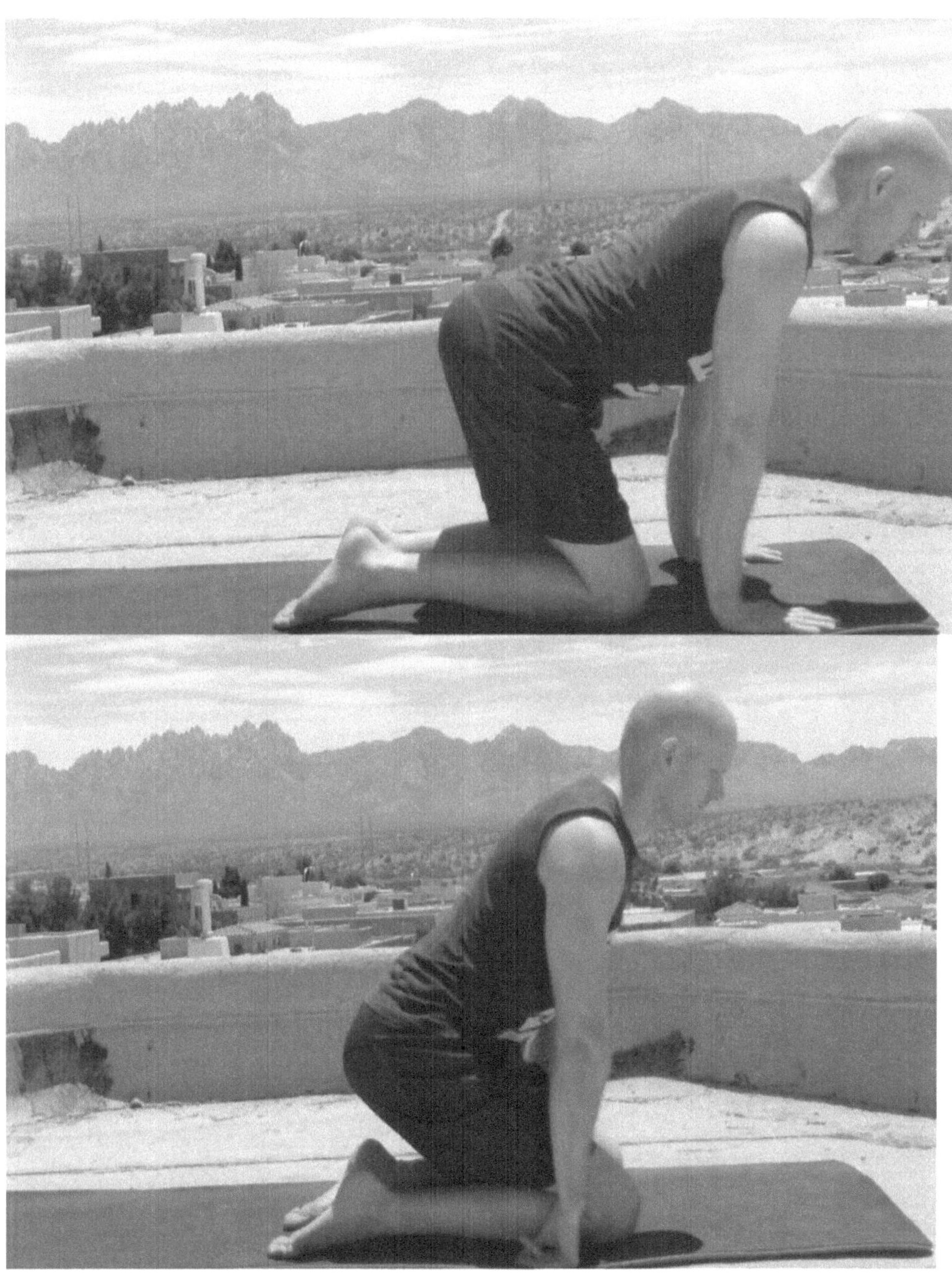

Ideally, you will eventually be able to sit your hips down between your heels:

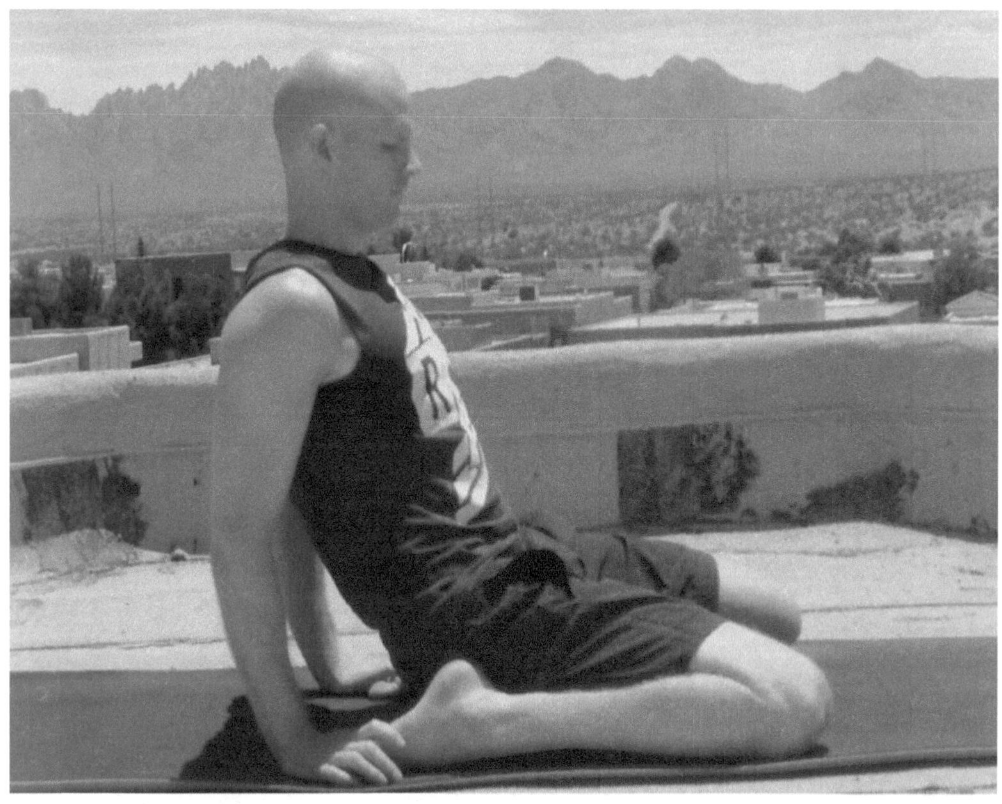

Then, if you're comfortable, you can drop back to your elbows:

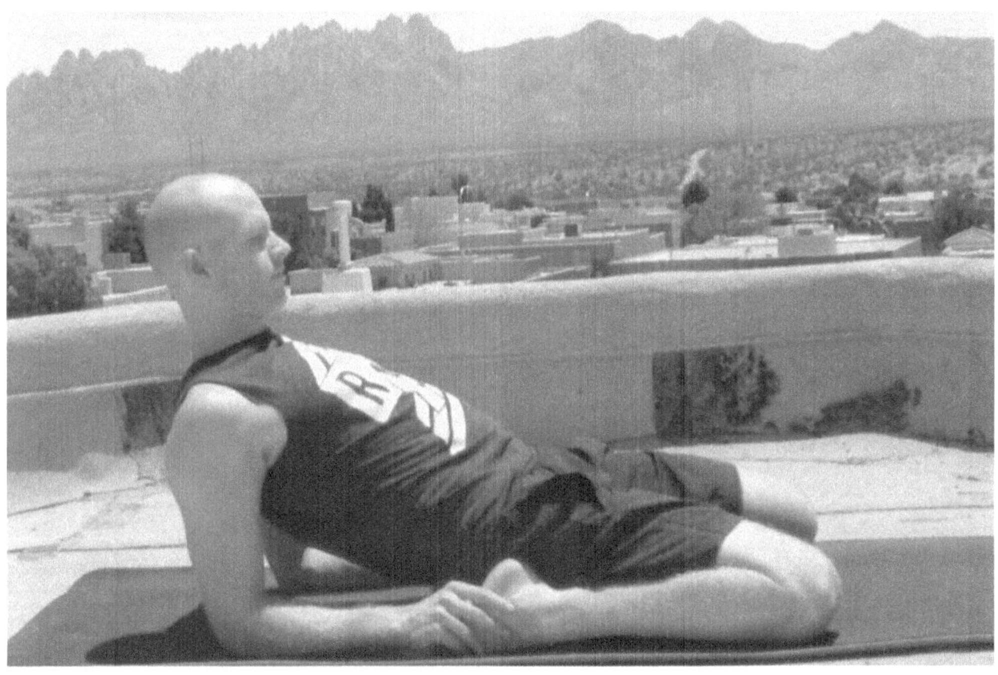

Lastly, you may drop your head back and take the opportunity to relax in this position for several rounds of breathing. Maintain a braced spine and a subtle lift in the chest. It can be helpful to think about squeezing your shoulder blades together here.

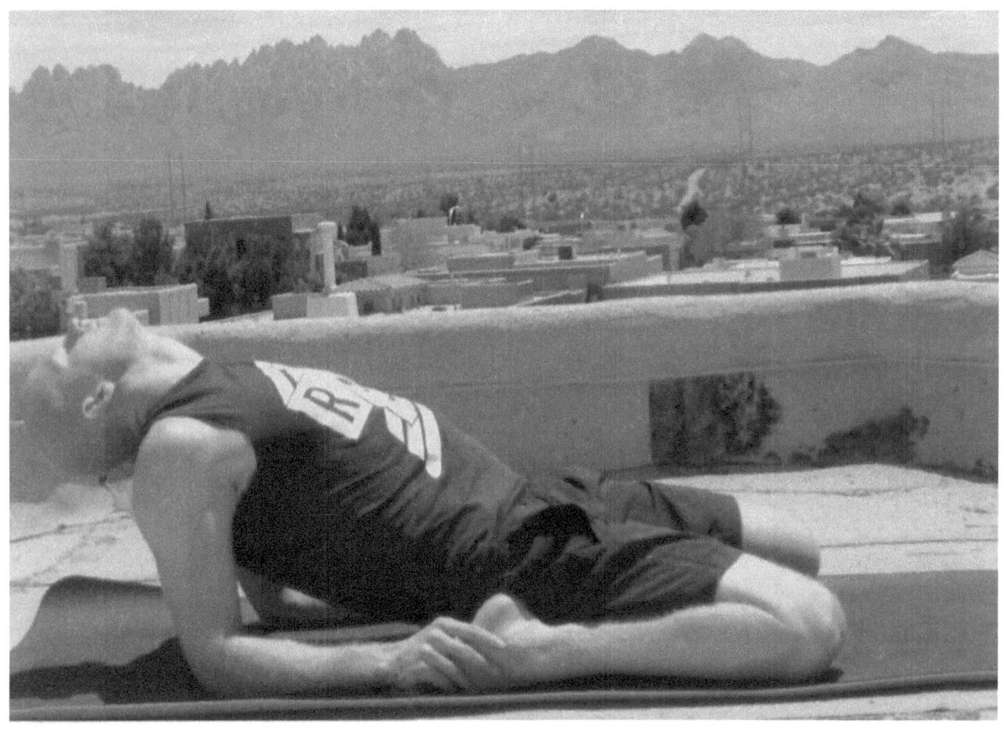

When you decide to reverse out of this position, please do so slowly, being **very careful** not to let your lower back collapse into flexion at any point along the way.

CHAPTER TWENTY-TWO

Meditation, Breath Awareness, and Finishing Your Practice

I like to end my practice by spending several minutes in Belly-Down Corpse Pose, meditating on my breath or simply scanning my body and noticing how I feel. If that version of the pose doesn't work for you, the more traditional Corpse Pose—lying on your back—works just as well.

Afterwards, I often take another few minutes to play around with my foam roller and my massage balls, to massage any 'tight spots' I noticed during my practice, whether it's my low back, my hips, my shoulders, hamstrings…whatever. If you enjoy self-massage, it's a nice way to 'reward' yourself for having finished your practice.

I have deliberately waited until the end of the book to mention the more meditative benefits you can derive from your home yoga practice, because I have found that for beginners it often adds an unnecessary element of distraction. The first step is to learn to really inhabit and listen to your body, and to simply breathe as calmly as possible during your practice. (In poses like the McGill Curl Ups or Turkish Get Ups, more vigorous breathing *is* often required, but mostly I coach students to breathe calmly and slowly through the nose.) But after you've figured out which postures work for you, establishing an ease with your practice and winding down your pain level, you may find that it's time to deepen your practice by giving more focus to the meditation aspect.

There are two ways to achieve this. You can either focus on the *length* of your breath—counting four or five seconds on the inhale, and the same on the exhale—or focusing on the *direction* of the breath. Or you can do both at once if you want more of a challenge! Focusing on the 'direction' of the breath is, dare I say, a little more 'woo woo,' as it involves picturing the *energy* of your breath traveling down your nose and into your belly on the inhale, and traveling back up your body and out of your nose on the exhale. It doesn't have to be some New Agey thing, though, and personally I just think of it as practicing my Jedi force powers.

It can be incredibly difficult to focus on maintaining perfect form *while* focusing on the breath, but the attempt can contract the mind wonderfully. You will notice that your focus drifts often—centering instead on anxieties, mundanities, life stressors, and so on—but all you have to do is gently nudge your focus back toward the breath, and you'll notice that your home yoga practice can flower, in tiny increments, into a home *meditation* practice as well.

I have designed this practice to be accessible to those students who are interested in the purely utilitarian pain-relieving and/or fitness aspects of the practice, but this other layer of the practice is always there to be discovered by those of you looking for something a little deeper.

I have discovered that there is no right or wrong way to go about a home yoga practice. There are no dogmas, no gurus, no egos, no competitions. In the absence of those distractions, it is my sincere hope that you can find the silence you need to listen to the wisdom of your body.

I hope you have found this book helpful, a gentle guide to finding your own spine-sparing home yoga practice, and I wish you the best on your continued healing journey.

-Justin